Rural Families and Reshaping Human Services

T0133626

This collection presents creative strategies and programs designed to address needs of families in the context of rural communities. Even before the most recent worldwide economic crisis, many rural families in the United States struggled to meet basic needs. As needs in rural communities have expanded, services have shrunk. This book identifies rural families' needs, including social supports during pregnancy, identification of adolescent risk behaviors, child safety, and basic services such as food and health care, using techniques such as Geographic Information Systems and needs and asset assessments. Strategies to address those needs include program development, the use of technology, and community partnerships.

The book reminds readers of the sense of independence and self-reliance found in many rural communities and the theme of diversity within rural communities runs throughout the book. The chapters are organized by identification of the needs of rural families, addressing disparities in rural areas, practice in rural communities, and human service organizations and professionals. Through research, practice, and creative works, the book contributes to a greater understanding of ways that service providers can advance their work with rural families and broaden their perspectives about realities experienced by families living in rural communities.

This book was originally published as a special issue of the *Journal of Family Social Work*.

Jeanne F. Cook, PhD, LISW-CP, has 25 years experience as a Social Worker in child welfare. She has been a social work educator since 1995 and joined the faculty at Johnson C. Smith University, USA, in 2011. In 2012, she was appointed as the Director of the JCSU MSW program.

Keith A. Alford, PhD, ACSW, Associate Professor, School of Social Work, Syracuse University, USA, is a former Treatment Foster Care Supervisor and Child Protective Services Worker. He has worked in human service agencies serving mid-western and southern rural communities. His research areas include family mental health and culturally specific programming.

Jennifer Uhrich, MPA, received her MPA from the University of Southern California, Sol Price School of Public Policy, USA, August 2014. She is currently an assistant editor of the *Journal of Family Social Work* and is an experienced qualitative researcher.

Pat Conway, PhD, LCSW, Senior Research Scientist, Essentia Institute of Rural Health, USA, is the editor of the *Journal of Family Social Work*. She conducts research regarding health, behavioral health and public health issues in rural and tribal communities.

Rural Families and Reshaping Human Services

Edited by
**Jeanne F. Cook, Keith A. Alford,
Jennifer Uhrich and Pat Conway**

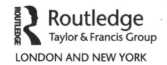
Routledge
Taylor & Francis Group

LONDON AND NEW YORK

First published 2015 by Routledge

2 Park Square, Milton Park, Abingdon, Oxon, OX14 4RN
605 Third Avenue, New York, NY 10017

Routledge is an imprint of the Taylor & Francis Group, an informa business

First issued in paperback 2020

Copyright © 2015 Taylor & Francis

British Library Cataloguing in Publication Data
A catalogue record for this book is available from the British Library

ISBN 13: 978-1-138-78792-6 (hbk)
ISBN 13: 978-0-367-73900-3 (pbk)

Typeset in ITC Garamond Light
by RefineCatch Limited, Bungay, Suffolk

Publisher's Note
The publisher accepts responsibility for any inconsistencies that may have
arisen during the conversion of this book from journal articles to book chapters,
namely the possible inclusion of journal terminology.

Disclaimer
Every effort has been made to contact copyright holders for their permission to
reprint material in this book. The publishers would be grateful to hear from any
copyright holder who is not here acknowledged and will undertake to rectify
any errors or omissions in future editions of this book.

Contents

CONTENTS

Rural Human Service Organizations and Providers

Citation Information

The following chapters were originally published in the *Journal of Family Social Work*. When citing this material, please use the original page numbering for each article, as follows:

Chapter 2
The Geography of Need: Identifying Human Service Needs in Rural America
Colleen Heflin and Kathleen Miller
Journal of Family Social Work, volume 15, issue 5 (November 2012) pp. 359–374

Chapter 3
Using GIS Mapping to Assess Foster Care: A Picture Is Worth a Thousand Words
Christine M. Rine, Jocelyn Morales, Anastasiya B.Vanyukevych, Emily G. Durand, and Kurt A. Schroeder
Journal of Family Social Work, volume 15, issue 5 (November 2012) pp. 375–388

Chapter 4
Changing Times in Rural America: Food Assistance and Food Insecurity in Food Deserts
Sarah Whitley
Journal of Family Social Work, volume 16, issue 1 (February 2013) pp. 36–52

Chapter 5
Rural Social Service Disparities and Creative Social Work Solutions for Rural Families Across the Life Span
Melinda L. Lewis, Diane L. Scott, and Carol Calfee
Journal of Family Social Work, volume 16, issue 1 (February 2013) pp. 101–115

Chapter 6
A Participant-Informed Model for Preventing Teen Pregnancy in a Rural Latino Community
Yvette Murphy-Erby, Kimberly Stauss, and Edwar F. Estupinian
Journal of Family Social Work, volume 16, issue 1 (February 2013) pp. 70–85

Chapter 15

Better Together: Expanding Rural Partnerships to Support Families
Harriet Shaklee, Jeri Bigbee, and Misty Wall
Journal of Family Social Work, volume 15, issue 5 (November 2012) pp. 389–400

Please direct any queries you may have about the citations to
clsuk.permissions@cengage.com

Introduction to Rural Families and Reshaping Human Services

JEANNE F. COOK

Johnson C. Smith University

KEITH A. ALFORD

School of Social Work, Syracuse University

JENNY UHRICH

Sol Price School of Public Policy, University of Southern California

PAT CONWAY

Essentia Institute of Rural Health

Myriad elements comprise the mosaic of diversity, including age, class, culture, disability, ethnicity, gender, gender identity and expression, immigration status, where one lives, nationality, race, religion, sex, sexual orientation, and political ideology. This book takes a look at one aspect of diversity that affects families and access to human services, living in rural areas. In a society inundated with social, familial, and economic challenges impacting the daily well-being of families, due diligence should be given to each sphere of human services. The contributors to this book have done just that, by focusing on rural America.

Prior to the most recent worldwide economic crisis beginning in 2008, many rural families in the United States struggled to meet their basic needs (Flynt, 1996; Stuart, 2004). Even in better economic times, rural families have had higher rates of unemployment and poverty compared to urban families (Economic Research Service, 2004; Flynt, 1996). In response, service providers in rural communities have had to use creative strategies, sometimes involving collaboration and cooperation among communities, to develop and deliver needed resources to families (Menanteau-Horta, 2005). Within the current economic and political environments, constraints on funding for services in rural communities have expanded, while need for services has grown. Programs have been combined, services reduced, and funding cut. At the same time, private non-profit agencies have seen donations shrink and client applications swell (Grant, 2010; Grenfeld, 2012; Pollack, 2011). Further complicating matters for rural family service provision, much of the current emphasis on where and how to cut services is based on the number of people served. As a result, rural programs, serving lower density populations, have been more severely impacted than urban communities.

Rural Families and Reshaping Human Services presents creative strategies and programs designed to address needs of families in the context of rural communities. It identifies rural families' needs, including social supports during pregnancy, identification of adolescent risk behaviors, child safety, and basic services such as food and health care, using techniques such as Geographic Information Systems and needs and asset assessments. Strategies presented to address those needs include program development, the use of new technologies, and community partnerships. Book chapters are organized by the needs of rural families; disparities in rural areas; practice with families in rural communities; and human service organizations and professionals in rural communities. Through research, practice, and creative works, the book broadens perspectives about realities experienced by families living in rural communities and contributes to a greater understanding of ways that service providers advance their work with rural families.

The chapters in this book address rural families at various stages of development (e.g., young children, adolescents, adults) from diverse backgrounds. The chapters describe diverse human service delivery systems, including health and behavioral health, prevention, and child welfare. Two chapters present technological innovations useful for better identification and understanding of needs in rural areas. This book examines challenges facing families in rural communities, along with innovative strategies to address those challenges. The chapters in this book highlight themes regarding assessment, needs and assets analysis, collaboration, social support, self-reliance, placement/locale, and cultural competency.

DEFINITIONS OF TERMS

Defining Rural

The US Census Bureau defines rural using classifications based on population density or population per square mile (http://www.census.gov/population/censusdata/urdef.txt). Urbanized areas include a central city and surrounding territory with a population of at least 50,000 and a population density of more than 1,000 people per square mile, including surrounding towns/places with a population of at least 2,500 people. Any area not meeting this definition is defined as rural.

The Office of Management and Budgets (OMB) utilizes counties instead of square miles as its unit of analysis. Counties designated as Metropolitan include an urban core area populated by at least 50,000 people. A Micropolitan area contains at least 10,000 (but less than 50,000) people. Counties not falling in either of these categories are designated as rural (Health Resources and Service Administration, 2012).

The Economic Research Service, United States Department of Agriculture, has developed two commonly used category schemes, the Rural-Urban Continuum Codes (RUCC) and the Rural-Urban Commuting Areas (RUCA) (http://www.ers.usda.gov/data-products/rural-urban-commuting-area-codes.aspx). The RUCC uses the Office of Management and Budget (OMB) metro and non-metro categories and subdivides them into three metro and six non-metro categories, resulting in a 9-part county codification (Economic Research Service, 2012). RUCA codes are based on zip codes, resulting in 10 major categories based on population density, urbanization, and daily commuting.

Methods for defining "rural" have remained diverse. Although Olaveson, Conway, and Shaver (2004) suggest that a universal definition of rural and its related concepts be adopted, this might be unrealistic. Having one definition for rural would allow comparison of research findings across studies. Public agencies would be better able to share data with each other, to more accurately determine overlaps and gaps in services, and to identify rural families' needs and strengths. On the other hand, differing methods of defining rural can be adapted for different purposes.

Defining Human Services

The National Association of Human Services provides the broadest definition of human services, as a variety of activities intended to meet human needs, prevent and remediate problems, and improve quality of life through an inter-disciplinary knowledge base (www.nationalhumanservices.org). Professionals and paraprofessionals deliver human services through public, private non-profit, and private for-profit sectors. Barker (2003) suggests that the terms human, social, and welfare services, can be used interchangeably, referring to any programs and services intended to enhance people's lives, development, and well-being. DiNitto (2011) defines social services as noneconomic services that provide care, counseling, education and other services.

Informal Resources

Informal resources, including neighbors, friends, and family, are the first line of defense for many rural families when they experience a crisis. This intrinsic support network may include church and civic memberships, reflecting long-term relationships (Barker, 2003; Watkins, 2005).

Defining Family

The U.S. Census Bureau defines family as "a group of two or more people who reside together and who are related by birth, marriage, or adoption" (http://factfinder2.census.gov/help/en/american_factfinder_help.htm#glossary/glossary.htm). By comparison, Barker (2003) suggests a broader definition of family, as individuals who assume some responsibilities for one another and live together. Although the typical American family is still often presented as two parents in their first marriage with children; families are diverse, including single parents with children, step-parent or blended families, families without children, families of diverse ethnicities and belief systems, multigenerational families in one household, individuals who come together by choice, and gay or lesbian couples (McGoldrick, Carter, & Garcia-Preto, 2012). The formation of families is often presented as a set of developmental stages that individuals go through, starting with single adults who join together as a couple, have and raise children, and face old age together (McGoldrick, Carter, & Garcia-Preto, 2012). Terkelson (1980) proposed that the process of caregiving for one another defines a family. Garland (2012) suggests that the processes that define family are identified by observation of behavior, including communication, shared meals and responsibilities, and provision of physical care.

RURAL FAMILIES AND THE CONTEXT OF PLACE: CHALLENGES, AND STRENGTHS

Challenges

Families living in rural communities may be challenged by the lack of availability of and access to resources, resulting from lack of funding, lack of transportation, and distance from service providers (Ashcraft, Owen, Braddock, Waring, & O'Bryant, 2009; Moore, 2008; Rodriguez, Mowrer, Romo, Aleman, Weffer, & Ortiz, 2010). Access to resources is particularly challenging for rural residents who are undocumented (Ashcraft, Owen, Braddock, Waring, & O'Bryant, 2009; Rodriguez, Mowrer, Romo, Aleman, Weffer, & Ortiz, 2010; Viramontez Anguiano & Lopez, 2012).

AVAILABILITY OF RESOURCES

Rural communities have less availability of social service, general health, and mental health resources. In a 2005 study, rural residents with HIV tended to have fewer outpatient visits and a reduced quality of health care compared to urban residents (Wilson, Korthuis, Fleishman, Conviser, Lawrence, Moore, & Gebo, 2011). King and Dabelko-Schoeny's (2009) qualitative study of rural Lesbian, Gay, Bisexual, and Transgender (LGBT) residents identified a lack of resource choices. A study of suicide rates among veterans found the lack of access to local mental health service providers to be a risk factor for rural veterans (McCarthy, Blow, Ignacio, Austin, & Valenstein, 2012). *New York Times* reporters Lowery and Pear (2012) suggest that increases in the population of older citizens and the extension of health care to more people through the Affordable Care Act will increase the number of potential patients in all areas of the United States, without a corresponding increase in the number of health care providers available. This will exacerbate the already existing higher than average median age and inadequate number of health care professionals in rural communities (Council of Economic Advisors, 2012).

DISTANCE FROM RESOURCES

Lack of transportation is particularly challenging for rural residents with disabilities, who are elderly, and/or who have health and mental health care needs (Transportation for America, 2010; McCarthy, Blow, Ignacio, Austin,

& Valenstein, 2012). King and Dabelko-Schoeny's (2009) qualitative study of middle age and older LGBT rural residents identified lack of transportation as a concern.

UNEMPLOYMENT AND POVERTY

At the height of economic expansion between 1991 and 2001, employment in rural communities was lower than in urban communities, 61.1% compared to 65.3%. By 2011, urban communities averaged a 59% employment rate, compared with 55% in rural communities, Male dominated industries and employment in the farming industries have been particularly hard hit by the economic downturn. (Economic Research Service, 2011; Freeland, 2012).

As employment opportunities declined from 2001 to 2011, the poverty rate rose. By 2009, the poverty rate had risen to 16.6% for nonmetropolitan populations, compared to the metropolitan area rate of 13.9% (Economic Research Service, 2011). In 2000 and 2009, the poverty rate for female-headed families in nonmetropolitan communities was 10% higher than for female-headed households in metro areas, growing from 37.1% in 2000 to 38.1% in 2009. The poverty rate for children in nonmetropolitan areas was 23.5% in 2009. (Economic Research Service, 2004, 2011; Mattingly & Stransky, 2010).

Strengths, Resiliency and Empowerment

Froma Walsh (2002) proposed that many families are resilient, with the capacity to successfully weather crises. Families who possess or develop more protective resources and have fewer risk factors are stronger or more resilient (Ganong & Coleman, 2002). One way to increase family resiliency is to identify existing family strengths and develop new ones (Saleeby, 2009). Towards that end, each chapter in this book contributes to a greater understanding of how service providers can advance their work with rural families, broadens their perspectives about realities experienced by families living in rural communities, and exhibits strategies utilized by rural families.

CHAPTER SUMMARIES

Each chapter in this book emphasizes the need for on-going attention to rural families and generates interest in the pursuit of more descriptive and investigative studies related to social work practice with rural families. Chapters offer tenets for best practice when working with rural families and reshaping rural human services. They are rich with insight and recommendations regarding dual relationships, caregiving for the young and the old, food assistance and insecurity, and health care. To pique readers' interest of what is to come, a synopsis of each chapter follows.

Rural Families and Their Needs

THE GEOGRAPHY OF NEED: IDENTIFYING HUMAN SERVICE NEEDS IN RURAL AMERICA
COLLEEN HEFLIN AND KATHLEEN MILLER, UNIVERSITY OF MISSOURI

Assessment in social work practice is on-going, as is refinement in assessment practices and tools. In *The Geography of Need: Identifying Human Service Needs in Rural America*, Colleen Heflin and Kathleen Miller present human service needs profiles as a method for understanding family needs in rural communities. After reviewing current methods for measuring level of rurality, Heflin and Miller propose using counties as the unit of analysis to determine need in counties that are significantly above the national average. Twelve indicators for demographic and economic needs are combined to create the human service needs profile. This model allows the graphic portrayal of needs within rural communities in order to identify risk factors and target special populations.

USING GIS MAPPING TO ASSESS FOSTER CARE: A PICTURE IS WORTH A THOUSAND WORDS
CHRISTINE M. RINE AND JOCELYN MORALES, PLYMOUTH STATE UNIVERSITY; ANASTASIYA
B.VANYUKEVYCH, NEW HAMPSHIRE DIVISION FOR CHILDREN, YOUTH AND FAMILIES;
EMILY G. DURAND AND KURT A. SCHROEDER, PLYMOUTH STATE UNIVERSITY

In keeping with the notion of needs identification, Christine Rine, Jocelyn Morales, Anastasiya Vanyukevych, Emily Durand and Kurt Schroeder use Geographic Information Systems (GIS) mapping to identify strengths and opportunities for improvement of New Hampshire's foster care system. In *Using GIS Mapping to Assess Foster Care: A Picture Is Worth a Thousand Words* the authors demonstrate mapping techniques that allow graphic depiction of child welfare. The innovation of GIS mapping has potential to expedite improvements in such key areas as transportation and school stability, two critical examples that speak to urgent needs of children in foster care. In addition, GIS mapping can be applied to other human service settings and other states with rural populations.

CHANGING TIMES IN RURAL AMERICA: FOOD ASSISTANCE AND FOOD INSECURITY IN
FOOD DESERTS
SARAH WHITLEY, WASHINGTON STATE UNIVERSITY

Food assistance for food insecure households is a concern in many rural settings. As such, it is an area *of* study that warrants attention. Sarah Whitley's qualitative chapter, *Changing Times in Rural America: Food Assistance and Food Insecurity in Food Deserts*, suggests that social integration and social capital are intertwined with food security in rural areas. Whitley's respondents, from an inland Washington county, share candid and sobering scenarios of their struggles and small victories over nutrition and limited food supply. Accounts of living in a food desert are shared and the logistics of food pantry operations are revealed.

Disparities and Rural Families

RURAL SOCIAL SERVICE DISPARITIES AND CREATIVE SOCIAL WORK SOLUTIONS FOR RURAL
FAMILIES ACROSS THE LIFE SPAN
MELINDA L. LEWIS AND DIANE L. SCOTT, UNIVERSITY OF WEST FLORIDA AND CAROL
CALFEE, SANTA ROSA COUNTY, FLORIDA

Melinda Lewis, Diane Scott and Carol Calfee's chapter, *Rural Social Service Disparities and Creative Social Work Solutions for Rural Families across the Life Span,* illustrates how collaborative partnerships in rural communities can effectively work together for the greater good. According to Lewis et al., "Social work in rural settings requires advanced generalist knowledge and skills to serve clients from birth to old age." Lewis et al. creatively share how various entities can come together to achieve a common goal, e.g., ameliorating rural homelessness. An interesting case study is presented in which the art of collaboration is explained.

A PARTICIPANT-INFORMED MODEL FOR PREVENTING TEEN PREGNANCY IN A RURAL
LATINO COMMUNITY
YVETTE MURPHY-ERBY, KIMBERLY STAUSS, AND EDWAR F. ESPUTINIAN, UNIVERSITY OF
ARKANSAS

A Participant-Informed Model for Preventing Teen Pregnancy in a Rural Latino Community, by Yvette Murphy-Erby, Kimberly Strauss, and Edwar F. Esputinian, walks the reader through the process of developing a culturally sensitive teen-pregnancy prevention program. This program is conceptualized by and for a rural Latino community. A thorough program description and highlights of its implementation contribute to the growing literature about the importance of cultural competency in rural communities.

Family Practice in Rural Communities

RURAL KINSHIP CAREGIVERS' PERCEPTIONS OF CHILD WELL-BEING: THE USE OF
ATTRIBUTION THEORY
RAMONA W. DENBY AND ALLISON BOWMER, UNIVERSITY OF NEVADA LAS VEGAS

Ramona W. Denby and Allison Bowmer's chapter, *Rural Kinship Care-givers' Perceptions of Child Well-Being: The Use of Attribution Theory,* examines variables associated with rural caregivers in their role of insuring the well-being of children. Attribution theory elucidates how people associate varying types of behaviors. The authors suggest that residents in rural communities, particularly small communities that are closely interconnected, may be less likely to be forthcoming about issues regarding children in their care. Rural families fear that their caretaker role may be called into question or perceived negatively. Caregivers were emboldened when they received social support from their community; essentially, having helpful friends and neighbors and knowing where and what outlets can be accessed make a positive difference toward optimal care provided to children by kinship families.

PREVENTING ADOLESCENT RISK BEHAVIOR IN THE RURAL CONTEXT: AN INTEGRATIVE
ANALYSIS OF ADOLESCENT, PARENT, AND PROVIDER PERSPECTIVES
CARRIE W. RISHEL, WEST VIRGINIA UNIVERSITY; LESLEY COTTRELL, WEST VIRGINIA
UNIVERSITY; AND TRICIA KINGERY, WEST VIRGINIA CHILD CARE ASSOCIATION

*Preventing Adolescent Risk Behavior in the Rural Context: An Integrative
Analysis of Adolescent, Parent, and Provider Perspectives*, examines perspectives of adolescents, parents, and providers regarding prevention of rural adolescent risk behaviors. Dispelling the myth that adolescents in rural settings do not engage in risky behavior, Rishel et al. purport that prevention efforts must include involvement of community residents, including parents, business leaders, and school and governmental personnel. The authors conclude that social workers must assess the needs of families, assess the needs of rural communities, and designate and train key stakeholders to mentor troubled youth.

RURAL WOMEN'S TRANSITIONS TO MOTHERHOOD: UNDERSTANDING SOCIAL SUPPORT
IN A RURAL COMMUNITY
CHRISTOPHER D. GJESFJELD, UNIVERSITY OF NORTH DAKOTA; ADDIE WEAVER, UNIVERSITY
OF MICHIGAN; AND KATHRYN SCHOMMER, THE VILLAGE FAMILY SERVICE CENTER

In *Rural Women's Transitions to Motherhood: Understanding Social
Support in a Rural Community,* Christopher D. Gjesfjeld, Addie Weaver, and Kathryn Schommer use the words of young women to illuminate realities of young mothers and their need for social support in rural settings. Becoming a mother may be viewed as a rite of passage for some, but when there is an absence of support and mentoring around expectations and means of survival, maternal distress can easily ensue. In the study, young women identified their partners and other women in their families as more important social supports than health care providers. Gjesfjeld et al. recommend that social workers tailor culturally-specific interventions and treatment plans to bolster informal support networks where needed.

INFLUENCING SELF-REPORTED HEALTH AMONG RURAL LOW-INCOME WOMEN THROUGH
HEALTH CARE AND SOCIAL SERVICE UTILIZATION: A STRUCTURAL EQUATION MODEL
TIFFANY BICE-WIGINGTON, STEPHEN F. AUSTIN STATE UNIVERSITY AND CATHERINE
HUDDLESTON-CASAS, UNIVERSITY OF NEBRASKA

In their chapter, *Influencing Self-Reported Health Among Rural Low-Income Women through Health Care and Social Service Utilization: A Structural Equation Model*, Tiffany Bice-Wigington and Catherine Huddleston-Casas illustrate the concept of intersetting knowledge through their study of rural women and access to health care. Using Structural Equation Modeling, the authors found that access to health care and social services was not correlated with better health outcomes. Intersetting knowledge, "an individual's ability to recall and apply information from one setting to another," was correlated with increased use of health care services.

FAMILY CAREGIVERS FOR SENIORS IN RURAL AREAS
DEBORAH J. MONAHAN, SYRACUSE UNIVERSITY

Deborah J. Monahan's conceptual chapter, *Family Caregivers for Seniors in Rural Communities*, enhances thinking around the complexities and realities of caring for the aged. She delineates elements associated with coping and burdens family caregivers experience. Monahan highlights several authors who demonstrate that reliance on religion acts as a protective function and steady resource for rural caregivers and the seniors they serve. A church or house of worship may sponsor senior-related activities and provide social service information. Monahan concludes, "While social workers may not be as comfortable asking questions about religious affiliation ... religious affiliation may be helpful in expanding services for rural caregivers." Monahan provides a canvas of the literature covering service needs, planning effective programs, access and barriers for rural caregivers, recent trends in caregiving, and the roles of social workers.

Rural Human Service Organizations and Providers

BAREFOOT, COUNTRY AND NAPPY: LIFE LESSONS OF A COLORED GIRL
NORA CHAMBERS CARTER, WINTHROP UNIVERSITY

Nora Chambers Carter's moving story of coming of age in a rural, southern community during a time of rapid social change is the focus of *Barefoot, Country and Nappy: Life Lessons of a Colored Girl*. She shares her personal challenges and resiliency, developed through her mother's teachings and her childhood community. Carter applies learning from her childhood to her present life and professional social work practice. She adeptly uses her own experiences to discuss access to social services, community support, and resiliency. Carter offers social workers another avenue for understanding challenges and resiliency unique to rural human services. The chapter illuminates the importance of using social workers' own experiences in effectively providing services, along with the importance of training to improve "cultural competency."

THE STRENGTHS OF RURAL SOCIAL WORKERS: PERSPECTIVES ON MANAGING DUAL RELATIONSHIPS IN SMALL ALASKAN COMMUNITIES
HEIDI BROCIOUS, JACQUELINE EISENBERG, JENNY YORK, HELEN SHEPARD, SHARON CLAYTON, AND BRITTANY VAN SICKLE, UNIVERSITY OF ALASKA FAIRBANKS

Maintaining allegiance to the profession's code of ethics is a routine task for service providers. The qualitative chapter, *The Strengths of Rural Social Workers: Perspectives on Managing Dual Relationships in Small Alaskan Communities*, by Heidi Brocious, Jacqueline Eisenberg, Jenny York, Helen Shepard, Sharon Clayton, and Brittany Van Sickle, explores the limitations of ethical codes in the context of dual relationships. Four salient themes emerge; rural social workers cannot avoid dual relationships, healthy dual relationships can be beneficial to clients, social work and other professional education make rural practice easier to negotiate, and rural social workers use complex critical thinking and develop advanced skills to negotiate dual relationships. Representative quotes enliven themes and provide depth around beliefs and understandings associated with the connection between dual relationships (between client and professional) and cultural competence. This research illuminates ways to make dual relationships work and provides concepts and processes applicable to other indigenous populations.

GIVING VOICE TO RURAL AND URBAN SOCIAL SERVICE PROVIDERS: RECESSIONARY EFFECTS ON THE PROVISION OF SERVICES IN HAWAI'I
REBECCA L. STOTZER AND CHRISTOPHER C.C. ROCCHIO, UNIVERSITY OF HAWAI'I

In the chapter, *Giving Voice to Rural and Urban Social Service Providers: Recessionary Effects on the Provision of Services in Hawai'i*, Rebecca Stotzer and Christopher Rocchio remind the reader that the economic downturn has greatly impacted those who live in and provide services for rural areas. Using quantitative and qualitative measures, the authors shed light on how the recession and budget crisis impacted the social service community within Hawai'i, a predominantly rural state. This chapter presents the views of social service supervisors, managers, and administrators serving rural clients. They candidly discuss realities of pay cuts and the need to close cases more quickly to keep case sizes manageable. Stotzer and Rocchio's discussion of provision of services under strict budgetary limitations is applicable to all social workers serving rural communities.

BETTER TOGETHER: EXPANDING RURAL PARTNERSHIPS TO SUPPORT FAMILIES
HARRIET SHAKLEE, UNIVERSITY OF IDAHO; JERI BIGBEE, UNIVERSITY OF CALIFORNIA, DAVIS; AND MISTY WALL, BOISE STATE UNIVERSITY

In *Better Together: Expanding Rural Partnerships to Support Families*, Harriet Shaklee, Jeri Bigbee, and Misty Wall suggest a multidisciplinary partnership between county extension educators, community health nurses, and social workers to better serve rural families. The authors demonstrate the advantages of this collaboration when serving grandparent caregivers in rural communities. Shaklee, Bigbee, and Wall highlight key problem areas and stressors (i.e., poverty, substance abuse, and financial stress) faced by families. These concerns are juxtaposed with key assets (i.e., cooperative extension programs, community health nurses, and prevention programs).

CONCLUSION

This book, dedicated to rural families, offers many critical initiatives worthy of emulation. Each chapter pinpoints pragmatic skills or salient points of interest that could be wisely employed by service providers. Knowledge building and knowledge sharing in social work remain essential elements for professional survival. The authors contributing to this book demonstrate new and revisited possibilities in rural America service provision that can serve as a springboard to future growth. Practitioners in the field can embrace noteworthy tenets outlined by the contributors to this book and begin to make inroads toward reshaping human services for rural families.

Almost three quarters of a century ago, Grace Abbott (1938) suggested that, to address current and future challenges to protect children, Americans should critically examine past steps, including the wrong turns taken because aims were unclear or fear of the unknown. Abbott's recommendation is as relevant today as when it was first written and can be applied to meeting the needs of rural families as well as their children. Chapters in this book describe past steps, current strategies, and recommendations for future actions, leading to lessons learned. Among the lessons identified for readers to take away are the following.

One Size does not Fit All

Currently, public policy tends to provide a limited number of opportunities for service delivery without consideration of the uniqueness of environment and how that might impact best practices. Rural human service providers can educate policy makers regarding policies that could be adapted to better meet the needs of individual rural communities, rather than forcing communities to adapt to a common set of criteria developed without regard for diversity.

Diversity is a Strength, not a Limitation

The mosaic of diversity in rural America brings strengths. When providers look at the differences represented among rural neighbors, they will discover a myriad of creative strategies that contribute to resiliency within and among rural families. These strategies can be incorporated into approaches implemented to address community needs. Rural families have a vested interest in the outcomes of policy and service decisions; they deserve to be represented around the tables where decisions are made.

Technology is One Solution for Increasing Access in Rural Communities

Emerging technologies offer creative possibilities for addressing some chronic problems in access to services in rural communities. Distance from providers can be eliminated through the availability of video conferencing, such as Skype. Other options to reduce isolation include Instagram, texting, and Facebook. As new advances occur and costs for technology decline, the list is endless.

The chapters in this book help point the way for solutions to current problems. As the twenty-first century progresses, new obstacles will be identified, offering new possibilities to discover the strengths, creativity, and resilience present in rural communities.

REFERENCES

Abbott, G. (1938). *The child and the state. (Vol. 1).* Chicago: University of Chicago Press.

Ashcraft, A., Owen, D., Braddock, E., Waring, S., & O'Bryant, S. (2009). Rural west Texans: Healthcare implications of "living the simple life." *Texas Public Health Journal, 61(1),* 8–12.

Barker, R. L. (2003). *The social work dictionary* (5th ed.). Washington, DC: NASW Press.

Council of Economic Advisors, Office of the President. (2012, June). *Strengthening the rural economy—The current state of rural America.* http://www.whitehouse.gov/administration/eop/cea/factsheets-reports/strengthening-the-rural-economy/the-current-state-of-rural-America

DiNitto, D. M. (2011). *Social welfare: Politics and public policy.* (7th ed.). Boston: Allyn & Bacon.

Economic Research Service. (2004). *Rural America at a glance.* Washington, DC: U.S. Department of Agriculture.

Economic Research Service. (2011). *Rural America at a glance.* Washington, DC: U.S. Department of Agriculture.

Economic Research Service. (2012). *Data for rural analysis.* Washington, DC: U.S. Department of Agriculture.

Flynt, W. (1996). Rural poverty in America. *National Forum, 76(3),* 32–35.

Freeland, C. (2012). The triumph of the family farm. *The Atlantic, 310(1),* 50–53.

Ganong, L. H., & Coleman, M. (2002). Family resilience in multiple contexts. *Journal of Marriage & Family, 64(2),* 346–348.

Garland, D. R. (2012). A process model of family formation and development. *Journal of Family Social Work, 15(3),* 235–250.

Grant, C. (2010). The spirit of child and youth care. *Relational Child and Youth Care Practice, 2(1),* 3–4.

Health Resources & Service Administration. (2012). *Defining the rural population.* Washington, DC: Author.

King, S., & Dabelko-Schoeny, H. (2009). "Quite frankly, I have doubts about remaining": Aging-in-place and health care access for midlife and older lesbian, gay, and bisexual individuals. *Journal of LGBT Health Research, 5(1-2),* 10–21.

Lowery, A., & Pear, R. (2012). Health law likely to make U.S. doctor shortage worse. *Charlotte Observer,* 23A.

Mattingly, M. J., & Stransky, M. L. (2010). *Child poverty in 2009: Rural poverty rate jumps to nearly 29 percent in second year of recession.* Durham, NH: Carsey Institute.

McCarthy, J. F., Blow, F. C., Ignacio, R. V., Austin, K. L., & Valenstein, M. (2012). Suicide among patients in the Veterans Affairs health system: Rural–urban differences in 275 rates, risks, and methods. *American Journal of Public Health,* 102, S111–S117.

McGoldrick, M., Carter, B., & Garcia-Preto, N. (2012). *Expanded family life cycle: Individual, family, and social perspectives* (4th ed.). New Jersey: Prentice Hall.

Menanteau-Horta, D. (2005). Strategies of cooperation and delivery of human services in rural areas: Sharing community assets. In L. Scales & C. Streeter (Eds.), *Rural social work: Building and sustaining community assets* (pp. 54–64). Belmont, CA: Brooks/Cole.

Moore, R. (2008). Rural women are at higher risk of blood pressure disorders during pregnancy. Paper presented at American Society of Nephrology's 41st Annual Meeting and Scientific exposition, Philadelphia, PA.

Olaveson, J., Conway, P., & Shaver, C. (2004). Defining rural for social work practice and research. In L. Scales & C. Streeter (Eds.), *Rural social work: Building and sustaining community assets* (pp. 9–20). Belmont, CA: Brooks/Cole.

Pollack, H. A. (2011). Health policy and the community safety net for people with disabilities. *Developmental Disabilities Research Reviews, 17*(1), 44–51.

Rodriguez, R., Mowrer, J., Romo, J., Aleman, A., Weffer, S. E., & Ortiz, R. M. (2010). Ethnic and gender disparities in adolescent obesity and elevated systolic blood pressure in a rural US population. *Clinical Pediatrics, 49*(9), 876–884.

Saleeby, D. (2009). *The strengths perspective in social work practice* (5th ed.). Boston, MA: Allyn & Bacon.

Stuart, P. H. (2004). Social welfare and rural people: From the colonial era to present. In L. Scales & C. Streeter (Eds.), *Rural social work: Building and sustaining community assets* (pp. 21–33). Belmont, CA: Brooks/Cole.

Terkelson, K. (1980). Toward a theory of the family life cycle. In E. A. Carter & M. McGoldrick (Eds.), *The family life cycle: A framework for family therapy* (pp. 21–52). New York, NY: Halsted Press.

Transportation for America. (2010, May 28). Panel examines rural transportation needs. *This Week in Washington*, 11–12.

U.S. Census Bureau. (2010). *Census urban and rural classification and urban area criteria*. Washington, DC: Author.

U.S. Census Bureau. (n.d.) *American fact finder*. Retrieved from http://factfinder2.census.gov/help/en/american_factfinder_help.htm#glossary/glossary.htm.

Viramontez Anguiano, R. P., & Lopez, A. (2012). El Miedo y El Hambre: Understanding the familial, social, and educational realities of undocumented Latino families in North Central Indiana. *Journal of Family Social Work, 15*(4), 321–336.

Walsh, F. (2002). A family resilience framework: Innovative practice applications. *Family Relations, 51*(2), 130–137.

Watkins, T. R. (2005). Natural helping networks: Assets for rural communities. In L. Scales & C. Streeter (Eds.), *Rural social work: Building and sustaining community assets* (pp. 65–76). Belmont, CA: Brooks/Cole.

Wilson, L. E., Korthuis, T., Fleishman, J. A., Conviser, R., Lawrence, P. B., Moore, R. D., & Gebo, K. A. (2011). HIV-related medical service use by rural-urban residents: A multistate perspective. *AIDS Care, 23*(8), 971–979. http://www.whitehouse.gov/administration/eop/cea/factsheets-reports/strengthening-the-rural-economy/the-current-state-of-rural-America.

The Geography of Need: Identifying Human Service Needs in Rural America

COLLEEN HEFLIN

Truman School of Public Affairs, University of Missouri, Columbia, Missouri

KATHLEEN MILLER

Rural Policy Research Institute, Truman School of Public Affairs, University of Missouri, Columbia, Missouri

Given the recent economic crisis and the accompanying funding cuts across social service programs, it is helpful to observe the geographic distribution of demographic characteristics and economic conditions that together create a human service needs profile. The authors provide a conceptual framework for a systematic analysis of county characteristics and demonstrate that rural areas of America have higher levels of needs and more complex needs than do metropolitan areas. This suggests that human service strategies that are successful in metropolitan areas may not translate well to nonmetropolitan areas.

The delivery of human services in America is undergoing a fundamental restructuring. The period of high unemployment rates, housing foreclosures, and poverty rates sometimes termed the "Great Recession" (Wessel, 2010) has created a historically high level of need for social services and strained the existing infrastructure. At the same time, state and federal budget deficits have resulted in deep cuts to basic social programs. Additionally, technological innovation has transformed the ways in which the public applies for and receives social services, as online application tools become more widespread for public safety net programs and telemedicine becomes more common in rural areas. Given these changes, it is of critical importance to understand the geographic distribution of human service needs to direct financial resources to targeted areas of need.

Fortunately, the need for information coincides with the first time release of American Community Survey (ACS) 5-year average county-level data by the U.S. Census Bureau in December 2010. Annual data are now released for counties with a population of 65,000 or more; 3-year average data is released for counties with population of 20,000 or more. Prior to this, data were only available for counties with populations above the 20,000 population threshold. Because data are currently available for each county in the United States, it is possible to conduct a comprehensive examination of human services need across the country. In this article, we describe a new place-based typology, which we call a "human service needs profile," that can be used to understand the unique social service challenges faced by rural America.

This article begins by describing the conceptual framework for existing place-based typologies and our rationale for creating a new typology built upon a human service needs profile. We then detail our data and methods for our typology, including a discussion of the relative trade-offs in using different geographic units of analysis. Results are shown for the human service needs typology for the nation as a whole and by rural county status. Tables and figures presented document how human service needs differ significantly, in the degree of need as well as the types of needs, in metropolitan and nonmetropolitan counties. In the conclusion, we discuss implications for policy and practice.

EXISTING PLACE-BASED TYPOLOGIES

There are numerous ways to categorize geography into different typologies based on the level of rurality of places. The most common typology is the Core Based Statistical Area (CBSA) designations by the Office of Management and Budget (2008), which categorizes counties into their official designation of metropolitan, micropolitan, and noncore. Counties that contain an urbanized area form the central counties of metropolitan areas, and surrounding counties that are linked through commuting ties are outlying counties of metropolitan areas. Counties that contain an urban cluster with between 10,000 and 49,999 individuals form the central counties of micropolitan areas, and surrounding counties that are linked through commuting ties are outlying counties of micropolitan areas. Counties not classified as metropolitan or micropolitan are considered noncore counties. Together, micropolitan and noncore counties make up nonmetropolitan counties and are usually equated with rural. Other typologies utilize the CBSA classifications as a basis but further divide these into additional categories based on the adjacency and size of urban place. The most common of these classifications are the

Rural-Urban Continuum Codes (RUCC) and the Urban Influence Codes developed by the Economic Research Service, U.S. Department of Agriculture (Economic Research Service, 2005).

One important consequence of the classification system for CBSAs is the inclusion of some very rural counties into metropolitan areas, due to the commuting criteria that links surrounding counties to metropolitan cores. There are 385 (35%) metropolitan counties that contain a population that is more than 50% rural. To address this issue, Isserman (2005) developed a county-level classification system that classifies counties based on the population density and distribution of population between urban and rural areas within the county, regardless of the CBSA status of the county. The resultant scheme is a simple four-level classification: urban, rural, mixed-rural, and mixed-urban.

County classifications remain a useful tool, given the availability of data with which to describe conditions and trends, but as is apparent from the previous classification schemes, it is difficult to classify counties into disparate groups. Recognizing this challenge, Waldorf (2007) developed the Index of Relative Rurality for all U.S. counties. This index is based on population, population density, extent of urbanized area, and distance to the nearest metropolitan areas. The index is scaled from 0 (*most urban*) to 1 (*most rural*).

Other typologies are not based solely on geography, but rather on economic and policy characteristics of rural America. The most common is the Economic Research Service (2005) county typologies, which seek to classify the United States based on the primary economic activity within each county in the United States (farming, mining, manufacturing, service, government, or nonspecialized). The policy typologies, which are not mutually exclusive, seek to identify particular characteristics that exist in geographic areas (persistent poverty, housing stress, low education, low employment, population loss, retirement destination, recreation).

Other typologies are more descriptive of the conditions in rural America. For example, Stauber (2001) divides rural America into four categories (urban periphery, sparsely populated, high amenity, high poverty). The Carsey Institute described "four rural Americas": amenity-rich, declining resource-dependent, chronically poor, and amenity/decline (Hamilton, Hamilton, Duncan, & Colocousis, 2008). Although all of these typologies provide a descriptive picture of rural America, none was designed to capture the full breadth of needs, which this analysis attempts to do.

RATIONALE FOR HUMAN SERVICE NEEDS PROFILE

Although growing academic thought has been devoted of late to the location of human services (Allard, 2009), not enough attention has been placed on the role of structural features of place such as population demographics and economic factors. Wolfe and Amirkhanyan (2010) took a step in this direction with their narrow exploration of the role of population aging on state and local expenditures. Larger studies of demographic change are not focused on the provision of human services directly, but on the shortage of managers in public organizations (Lew & Cho, 2011) or managing diversity in the workplace (Broadnax, 2010). Given the wide variation of programs and services that fall under the large umbrella of "human services," an effort to try to identify the magnitude of needs across the life course at the geographic level requires a multidimensional approach. As a consequence, the development of a human service needs profile was informed by an understanding of how population demographics combine with economic risk factors to create different patterns of need across the country. This section contains the rationale for our approach.

Human service needs depend on the characteristics of the population in need. For example, elderly populations require different programs and services to meet their needs than do households with young children. Similarly, as compensation for military service, veterans have access to a host of programs and services that are not available to non-veteran households. In these instances, the human service needs of an area will depend upon the age structure, fertility rate, and prevalence of veterans in the population.

Additionally, the provision of human services may need to be adapted to deal with language barriers, cultural issues, transportation needs, or low education levels. For example, human service providers in areas with a high foreign born population may find it helpful to provide services in languages besides English. Culturally appropriate programming may be needed in areas with high levels of Native American or Hispanic populations. In areas with high levels of transportation barriers, it may be necessary for service providers to adopt online approaches to service delivery. Conversely, in areas in which a high proportion of the population lacks a high school diploma, online approaches to service delivery may be more challenging.

Human services needs are also partly a function of the economic needs of an area. There is a long history of identifying the needs of an area by focusing on the proportion of the area that is poor and the percent of total income received from government transfers. More recently, the Supplemental Nutritional Assistance Program (SNAP; formerly known as Food Stamps) participation rate has become an alternative measure of economic distress (Slack & Myers, 2012). The economic distress of the recent recession has led to family distress, as evidenced by the increase in multifamily households (Mykyta & Macartney, 2011).

SELECTING THE UNIT OF ANALYSIS

In selecting geographic units for analysis below the state level, there are relatively few standard statistical units to choose between: counties, public-use micro data areas (PUMAs), census tracks, and census-block groups.

- Counties provide an easily recognized unit of analysis that is stable over time, with few exceptions. Although counties are not often recognized as an official unit of government in New England states (Connecticut), data is still tabulated at that level in other states across the United States and is readily available from several sources such as the U.S. Departments of Labor, Agriculture and Health and Human Services.
- Public use micro data areas (PUMAS) are geographic areas developed by the Census Bureau for which raw data is provided. The geographic size of a PUMA varies widely, based on population, but each PUMA has approximately 100,000 population. However, the geographic boundaries of PUMAS change over time.
- A Census tract is a subdivision of counties that contain between 1,500 and 8,000 people, with the optimal size being 4,000. The geographic size of tracts varies widely, depending on the density of population.
- A Census-block group has a population of 300 to 6,000, with the optimal size being 1,500. These are the lowest geographic unit for which the Census Bureau tabulates and presents data in the ACS.

Of the four statistical units, only counties are consistent over time and provide geographic boundaries that also correspond to meaningful political boundaries. As a result, we use the county as the main unit for our analysis. The disadvantage to this approach is that the size of counties is not homogenous across the United States, resulting in modifiable areal unit problem (see Heywood, Cornelius, & Carver, 1998; Taylor, Gorard, & Fritz, 2003). In general, counties tend to be smaller in the East and larger in the West. Because of the size differential, counties in the East are more likely to be homogeneous than counties in the West. Western counties therefore may have pockets of need that are of similar size to pockets of need in the East, but because the pockets are contained within larger geographic units, the need is not identified by our method here. Although this possibility is more prevalent in larger geographic counties such as in the West, this does occur across all states and is the same problem that is inherent with other official statistics such as county unemployment rates, poverty rates, and the like. Though counties are not ideal, they are the best unit available for our purposes.

County-level data come from Census Bureau Annual Population Estimates (U.S. Census Bureau, Population Division, 2010), the Census Bureau ACS 5-year average data (U.S. Census Bureau, 2010a), the Census Bureau Small Area Income and Poverty Estimates (U.S. Census Bureau, 2010b), the Bureau of Economic Analysis Regional Economic Information System (Bureau of Economic Analysis, 2010), and the Veteran's Administration (2010). From Annual Population Estimates, we calculate the percent of the population age 65 and older and the percent of the population that is Native American, Hispanic, and African American. The work dependency ratio is calculated as the ratio of the population younger than age 20 and older than 64 to the population age 20 to 64. The percent of the population that are veterans is based on county-level estimates from the Veteran's Administration divided by the total population from the Population Estimates.

We use data from the ACS 2005–2009 5-year county-level averages for data on the percentage of the county population in subfamilies, the number of births to women age 15 to 50, the percentage of the population age 25 and older without a high school diploma, the percentage of the population that is foreign born, the percentage of households without a vehicle available, and the percent of households participating in SNAP. Finally, the county-level poverty rate comes from the Small Area Income and Poverty Estimates (SAIPE) from the Census Bureau. County-level data on the percent of total county income from transfers is taken from the BEA REIS for 2008.

Because the use of a 5-year average data point may smooth out trends in specific indicators, we utilized annual data wherever available for counties as an alternative to the ACS. The official counts of population from the Census Bureau are the annual population estimates, so this is the proper source for the age, race, and ethnicity calculations. The annual data estimates for poverty were selected over the 5-year average to avoid the smoothing out of the poverty that may result from including the prerecession years in the average. For several indicators, however, the ACS is the only available source for data. Although ACS data are available at an annual basis and 3-year average for some counties, the 5-year average data are used for all counties for consistency's sake.

For each measure, we examined the national county-level distribution and selected the 90th percentile as the threshold that indicates that the county has a need that is significantly above the national average. Additionally, this decision rule provides a consistent number of counties in each of the need indicators, which has the side benefit of assigning equal weight to each need indicator in the total human service needs profile; approximately 314 counties are defined as having a high level of need for each of the measures. Although using the 90th percentile as the cut-off has the advantage that it is a consistent rule, it does have several limitations. In some cases, the number of counties with a recognized need is actually higher than the 314 that we allow. This is the case for poverty, in which a high-poverty county is often defined as a county with a poverty rate above 20% (Economic Research Service, 2005). Using the 90th percentile rule, however, results in a threshold of 25%. In other cases, the 90th percentile rule may be too generous. For example, in the case of Native Americans, the 90th percentile rule results in a threshold of 3% of the total population. In most cases, however, the rule results in a substantively meaningful threshold.

DEMOGRAPHIC NEEDS PROFILE

To begin, eight indicators were selected that summarize the demographic characteristics of the population at a county level (see Table 1). Indicators represent human services needs of individuals across the life course from infancy to old age (percent of the population age 65 and older, the number of births to women age 15 to 50, and the work-age dependency ratio). Counties are identified as having a human service need if they have a high Native American, Hispanic, or African American population. To capture the human capital level of the area, the percent of the population age 25 and older without a high school diploma is included. The proportion of the population that are veterans and the proportion of the population foreign born are included to provide insight into specialized service needs. Finally, a measure of the percent of the population living in subfamilies is included to capture different family living arrangements, a potential factor in designing treatment interventions.

Next, we present the summation of demographic needs by county type (metropolitan, micropolitan, and noncore counties) (see Table 2). Counties receive one "point" for each area in which they exceed the 90th percent

TABLE 1 Demographic Needs Profile

Indicator	National Average (%)	90th Percentile (%)	Data Source
Percent of population age 65 and older	12.9	21.0	Census Bureau Population Estimates, 2009
Racial/ethnic minorities			
African American	12.9	30.0	Census Bureau
Native American	1.0	3.0	Population Estimates,
Hispanic/Latino	15.8	21.0	2009
Percent of population living in subfamilies	3.0	5.0	American Community Survey, 2005–2009
Work age dependency ratio (Population younger than age 20 and older than age 64 to Population 20 to 64)	66.8	87.0	Census Bureau Population Estimates, 2009
Birth to women age 15 to 50	5.6	8.0	American Community Survey, 2005–2009
Veterans as percent of total population	7.4	12.0	Census Bureau Population Estimates, 2009; Veterans Administration, 2009
Percent of population age 25 and over without a high school diploma	15.4	28.0	American Community Survey, 2005–2009
Percent of population foreign born	12.4	10.0	American Community Survey, 2005–2009

national distribution. Each counties' demographic needs profile is created by summing the demographic needs over all eight measures. Although 45.8% of U.S. counties have no demographic characteristics that exceed the 90th percentile for all U.S. counties, 25% are identified by a single demographic need, 16.5% have two demographic needs, 7.5% have three demographic needs, and 3.8% of counties have four or more demographic needs. No county has all eight demographic needs; the highest number of demographic needs observed jointly is seven, which is found in Hall County, Texas.

Although just over one-half of all counties experience at least one of the risk factors, these counties are clustered in the middle of the country in largely continuous patterns stretching along Iowa, Illinois, Wisconsin, Michigan, Indiana, Ohio, Pennsylvania, New York, New Hampshire, Vermont, and Maine (see Figure 1). It is important to note that when areas do not show up as having high demographic needs, it does not indicate that there are not important demographic issues that shape human service delivery in a county. Instead, the issues in these counties are not noteworthy in a national analysis of areas with high needs. In contrast, areas with three or more risk factors are concentrated in several geographic regions of the country: the Mississippi Delta, Texas border region, Central California, Great Plains, and areas with high Native American populations.

It is clear that high demographic need counties are overrepresented among noncore and micropolitan counties (see Table 2). Although only 31.1% of noncore counties have no demographic needs, 58.3% of metropolitan counties and 54.8% of micropolitan counties fall into this category. In fact, noncore and micropolitan counties are more likely to have each nonzero level of demographic needs than metropolitan areas. For example, though 3.3% of metropolitan counties have three demographic needs, 5.7% of micropolitan and 11.9% of noncore counties have the same. Thus, the data indicate that rural areas are much more likely to have demographic characteristics that are suggestive of high human service needs.

TABLE 2 Demographic Needs Summary by County Type

Number of Demographic Risk Factors	Metropolitan		Micropolitan		Noncore		All Counties	
	n	%	n	%	n	%	n	%
0	641	58.3	376	54.8	422	31.1	1,439	45.8
1	275	25.0	155	22.6	399	29.4	829	26.4
2	129	11.7	91	13.3	300	22.1	520	16.5
3	36	3.3	39	5.7	162	11.9	237	7.5
4	15	1.4	17	2.5	56	4.1	88	2.8
5	2	0.2	5	0.7	14	1.0	21	0.7
6	2	0.2	3	0.4	3	0.2	8	0.3
7	0	0.0	0	0.0	1	0.1	1	0.0
8	0	0.0	0	0.0	0	0.0	0	0.0

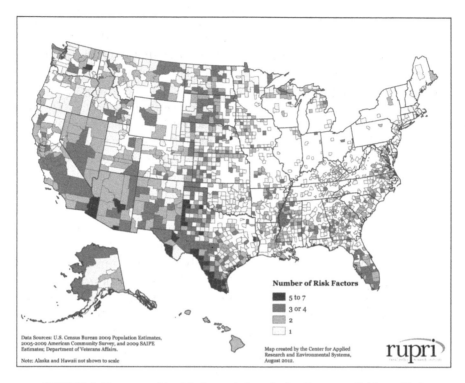

FIGURE 1 Demographic risk factor index. (color figure available online)

ECONOMIC NEEDS PROFILE

Next, measures that describe the economic structure of a county were considered. The economic needs included in the needs profile were the poverty
rate, the percentage of housing units with no transportation (Dabson,
Johnson, & Fluharty, 2011), the percentage of the household receiving SNAP
benefits, and the percentage of the total county income that is received from
transfer payments (see Table 3). We excluded the county unemployment rate
because of the very high correlation with the poverty rate. Interestingly,
SNAP participation and total income from transfer payments are not highly
correlated, largely as a result of wide statewide variation in disability, Unemployment Insurance and Temporary Assistance for Needy Families (TANF)
program receipt. SNAP is included separately because it is the only program
with eligibility guidelines that are regulated at the federal level.

As with the demographic needs profile, counties with economic characteristics above the 90th percent national distribution receive one point for
each area in which they exceed the threshold (see Table 4). The economic
needs profile is computed by summing the index of economic needs across
the four measures: more than three-fourths of all counties have no economic
needs identified, 12.6% have one economic need, 4.4% have two economic

TABLE 3 Economic Needs Profile

Indicator	National Average (%)	90th Percentile (%)	Source
County poverty rate for total population	14.2	25.0	Census Bureau Small Area Income and Poverty Estimates, 2009
Percent of housing units with no vehicles available	8.8	10.0	American Community Survey, 2005–2009
Percent of households receiving Supplemental Nutritional Assistance Program benefits	8.5	18.0	American Community Survey, 2005–2009
Percent of total county income from transfer payments	15.3	32.0	Bureau of Economic Analysis, Regional Economic Information System, 2008

needs, 3.8% have three economic needs, and 2.0% have four economic needs. The experience of multiple economic risk factors is concentrated in Appalachia, the black belt, Mississippi Delta, Texas border region, and areas with high Native American populations (see Figure 2). Although the Economic Risk Factor Index offers few surprises on its own as the highlighted regions are often considered areas of economic distress, it is helpful to observe how the areas of economic need differ from those with demographic needs.

Finally, the distribution of economic needs by the rurality of the county once again demonstrates that high areas of need are concentrated in nonmetropolitan areas of the country. Although 85.2% of metropolitan areas have no economic need, only 78.9% of micropolitan and 69.9% of noncore score the same (see Table 4). Fourteen and one-half percent of noncore counties have one economic need, compared to 11.4% of micropolitan and 11.0% of metropolitan counties. Six and one-half percent of noncore counties have two economic needs, compared to 3.4% of micropolitan and 2.5% of metropolitan. Only one metropolitan county scores high on all four economic

TABLE 4 Economic Needs Summary by County Type

Number of Economic Risk Factors	Metropolitan		Micropolitan		Noncore		All Counties	
	n	%	n	%	n	%	n	%
0	937	85.2	541	78.9	949	69.9	2,427	77.2
1	121	11.0	78	11.4	197	14.5	396	12.6
2	28	2.5	23	3.4	88	6.5	139	4.4
3	13	1.2	31	4.5	74	5.5	118	3.8
4	1	0.1	13	1.9	49	3.6	63	2.0

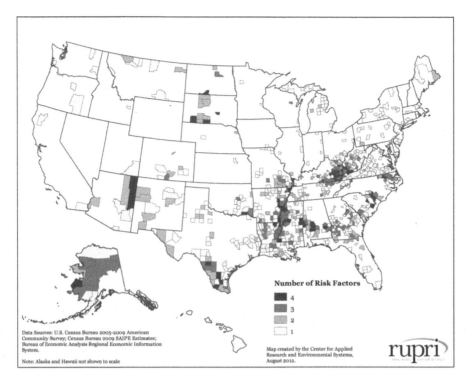

FIGURE 2 Economic risk factor index. (color figure available online)

measures, but 13 micropolitan counties and 49 noncore counties meet the same criteria. Thus, it is clear that high economic need counties are more heavily concentrated in noncore and micropolitan counties than in metropolitan areas.

HUMAN SERVICE NEEDS PROFILE

Because economic and demographic needs together structure human service needs, demographic and economic needs profiles are combined to create a human service need profile across the eight demographic and four economic measures, totaling 12 potential needs (see Table 5). When economic and demographic factors are considered together, the majority of counties are identified by scoring in the top 90th percentile on at least one measure; only 40.6% of all counties do not have any needs measure. Just less than one-fourth of counties have a single human service need, with the remaining one-third of all counties having multiple or co-occurring human service needs. Note that no county is observed to have more than nine human service needs co-occurring at one time; the five counties with the highest number of human service needs present are all in Texas (Brooks, Hall, Maverick, Starr, & Zavala Counties).

TABLE 5 Combined Human Services Needs Summary by County Type

Number of Risk Factors	Metropolitan		Micropolitan		Noncore		All Counties	
	n	%	*n*	%	*n*	%	*n*	%
0	585	53.2	335	48.8	355	26.2	1,275	40.6
1	267	24.3	149	21.7	315	23.2	731	23.3
2	149	13.5	83	12.1	263	19.4	495	15.7
3	51	4.6	42	6.1	174	12.8	267	8.5
4	29	2.6	34	5.0	120	8.8	183	5.8
5	11	1.0	15	2.2	74	5.5	100	3.2
6	4	0.4	18	2.6	27	2.0	49	1.6
7	2	0.2	8	1.2	15	1.1	25	0.8
8	2	0.2	0	0.0	11	0.8	13	0.4
9	0	0.0	2	0.3	3	0.2	5	0.2

Areas with comorbid human service needs are scattered throughout the country, with concentrations occurring in some expected locations such as the Texas border region, the Delta, the Ozarks, and Appalachia (see Figure 3). However, some geographic regions highlighted by this analysis are less expected, such as southern Florida, the group of counties in northwest Texas, the large number of counties in the upper Great Plains

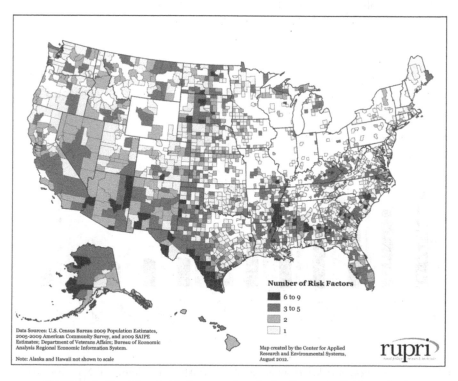

FIGURE 3 Combined risk factor index. (color figure available online)

and eastern Montana, and counties in northern Michigan. Once again, the center of the country from Iowa up to Maine is noted by the lack of critical needs.

As with demographic and economic needs alone, areas with higher levels of need on the human service needs profile are overrepresented in micropolitan and noncore counties. Nearly one-half of all metropolitan counties have no risk factors, whereas only one-fourth of noncore counties have none. In fact, as the number of risk factors increases beyond one, the greater the likelihood that a county will be noncore or micropolitan rather than metropolitan. This again suggests that the complexity of the human service needs in nonmetropolitan areas is much greater than in metropolitan areas.

To ground the discussion of exactly how human service needs differ in metropolitan and nonmetropolitan areas, we present a comparison of the human service needs that occur in isolation by county metropolitan status (nonmetropolitan combines micropolitan and noncore counties) (see Figure 4). Looking only at one-fourth of all counties that have a single risk factor, it is clear that metropolitan and nonmetropolitan counties differ significantly in terms of the types of human service needs that are present. For example, of all counties that score in the top decile of the distribution on share of total population that are veterans, 27% of nonmetropolitan and 55% of metropolitan counties have no other risk factor present.

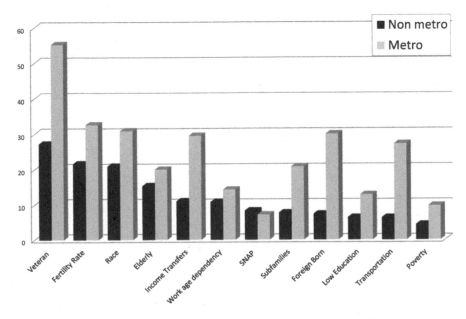

FIGURE 4 Occurrence of risk factors alone. *Note.* SNAP = Supplemental Nutrition Assistance Program.

First, in each case, the bars are higher for metropolitan counties than they are for nonmetropolitan counties, with the lone exception of SNAP receipt. This indicates that human service needs are less likely to occur in isolation in nonmetropolitan areas than they are in metropolitan areas. This is significant because counties with a single human service need can focus more narrowly on meeting the needs of that single population, whereas counties that score in the top decile across multiple categories have a more complex set of issues to address.

It is also apparent that the rankings of human service needs differ in metropolitan and nonmetropolitan areas. Although high-veteran populations, high racial minority populations, and high-fertility counties are the three most common human service needs to occur alone in metropolitan and nonmetropolitan areas, the relative importance of the different human service needs is very different for the other nine human service needs. For example, though having a high percentage of foreign born populations present is ranked ninth for nonmetropolitan areas, it is ranked fourth for metropolitan areas. Once again, these differences suggest that approaches that work well in metropolitan areas may not translate well to nonmetropolitan counties.

SUMMARY AND CONCLUSIONS

Given the recent economic crisis and the accompanying funding cuts across social service programs, it is helpful to observe the geographic distribution of demographic characteristics and economic conditions that together structure the human service needs profile. Guided by the recognition that demographic characteristics and economic conditions play a critical role in shaping the human service needs at the county level, a systematic analysis demonstrates that rural areas of America have high levels of needs and more complex needs than do urban areas.

Limitations

This approach is not without its limitations. Choosing counties as the geographic unit is problematic because counties are larger in the West than in the rest of the United States. However, this limitation is also present with other available geographic units, such as PUMAs, census tracts, or block groups. Counties have the advantage of often being coterminous with human service delivery boundaries. Another limitation is the choice of the 90th percentile as a cut-point. However, we have tested our analysis with other cut-points, such as the 80th percentile and with standardized measures, and our conclusions remain unchanged: Nonmetropolitan areas score higher on this human service needs profile than do metropolitan areas.

Conclusion

Given the rapid transition in the demand and supply of human services in this country, a "one-size-fits-all" approach to human service delivery is no longer appropriate. We have demonstrated the geographic distribution of counties with high levels of human service needs, as defined by the top 10 percentile ranking of all counties for the eight demographic and four economic risk factors. The type and number of risk factors present in metropolitan and nonmetropolitan counties differ substantially, with nonmetropolitan counties more likely to have multiple risk factors present. This suggests that human service strategies that are successful or prioritized in metropolitan areas may not translate well to nonmetropolitan areas. Additionally, a need for integrated human service delivery may be even more critical in nonmetropolitan areas than metropolitan areas.

We hope that this development of a conceptual framework to identify a county-based human service needs profile can be improved by other researchers and utilized by policy makers and practitioners. Given the limited human service funds available, it is more important now than ever to be mindful of the demographic and economic contours in which services are being provided.

REFERENCES

Allard, S. (2009). *Out of reach: Place, poverty, and the new American welfare state.* New Haven, CT: Yale University Press.

Broadnax, W. D. (2010). Diversity in public organizations: A work in progress. *Public Administration Review, 70*(Issue Suppl.), s1177–s179.

Bureau of Economic Analysis. (2010). *Regional Economic Information System, 2008.* Retrieved from http://www.bea.gov/regional/index.htm

Dabson, B., Johnson, T. G., & Fluharty, C. W. (2011, April). *Rethinking federal investments in rural transportation: Rural considerations regarding reauthorization of the Surface Transportation Act* (RUPRI Rural Policy Brief). Columbia, MO: Rural Policy Research Institute, Truman School of Public Affairs.

Economic Research Service. (2005). *USDA measuring rurality briefing room.* Retrieved from http://www.ers.usda.gov/Briefing/Rurality/Typology/

Hamilton, L. C., Hamilton, L. R., Duncan, C. M., & Colocousis, C. R. (2008). Place matters: Challenges and opportunities in four rural Americas. *Carsey Institute Report on Rural America, 1*(4).

Heywood, I., Cornelius, S., & Carver, S. (1998). *An introduction to geographical information systems.* New York, NY: Addison Wesley Longman.

Isserman, A. M. (2005). In the national interest: Defining rural and urban correctly in research and public policy. *International Regional Science Review, 28*(4), 465–499.

Lew, G., & Cho, Y. J. (2011). The aging of the state government workforce: Trends and implications. *American Review of Public Administration, 42*(1), 48–60.

Mykyta, L., & Macartney, S. (2011). *The effects of recession on household composition: "Doubling up" and economic well-being* (U.S. Census Bureau SEHSD Working Paper No. 2011–4). Washington, DC: Poverty Statistics Branch, U.S. Census Bureau.

Office of Management & Budget. (2008, November 20). *Update of statistical area definitions and guidance on their uses* (OMB Bulletin 09–01). Washington, DC: Executive Office of the President, Office of Management and Budget.

Slack, T., & Myers, C. (2012). Understanding the geography of food stamp participation: Do space and place matter? *Social Science Research, 41*, 263–275.

Stauber, K. N. (2001). *"Why invest in rural America – And how? A critical public policy question for the 21st Century." Exploring policy options for a new Rural America.* Center for the Study of Rural America, Federal Reserve Bank of Kansas City.

Taylor, C., Gorard, S., & Fritz, J. (2003). The modifiable areal unit problem: Segregation between schools and levels of analysis. *International Journal of Social Research Methodology, 6*(1), 41–60.

U.S. Census Bureau. (2010a). *American Community Survey 2005–2009 five year estimates.* Retrieved from http://factfinder2.census.gov/faces/nav/jsf/pages/index.xhtml

U.S. Census Bureau. (2010b). *Small area income and poverty estimates, state and county estimates for 2008.* Retrieved from http://www.census.gov/did/www/saipe/data/statecounty/data/2008.html

U.S. Census Bureau, Population Division. (2010). *Annual estimates of the resident population by age, sex, race and Hispanic origin for counties in [state]: April 1, 2000 to July 1, 2009.* Retrieved from http://www.census.gov/popest/data/historical/2000s/vintage_2009/datasets.html

Veteran's Administration. (2010). *County level veteran population by state: 2000–2030.* Retrieved from http://www.va.gov/vetdata/Veteran_Population.asp

Waldorf, B. (2007). Measuring rurality. *InContext, 8*(1). Bloomington, IN: Indiana Business Research Center, Indiana University.

Wessel, D. (2010). Did "great recession" live up to the name? *The Wall Street Journal.* Retrieved from http://online.wsj.com/article/SB10001424052702303591204575169693166352882.html

Wolf, D., & Amirkhanyan, A. (2010). Demographic change and its public sector consequences. *Public Administration Review, 70*, S12–S23.

Using GIS Mapping to Assess Foster Care: A Picture Is Worth a Thousand Words

CHRISTINE M. RINE and JOCELYN MORALES

Plymouth State University, Plymouth, New Hampshire

ANASTASIYA B. VANYUKEVYCH

New Hampshire Division for Children, Youth and Families, Concord, New Hampshire

EMILY G. DURAND and KURT A. SCHROEDER

Plymouth State University, Plymouth, New Hampshire

Geographic Information Systems (GIS) have become widely used outside of traditional mapping applications, expanding their reach to social service organizations. The purpose of this article is to describe and explore the benefits of GIS mapping in identifying strengths and needs of foster care systems in rural settings through graphically assessing service usage and delivery. Herein, authors present their project as an example of such efforts to inform applications for practice providing a model that encourages others to explore methods of this nature. Focus is placed on rural characteristics that bring particular challenges for child welfare stakeholders.

This article explores the utility of mapping to better understand service usage and delivery for foster care youth. Specifically, the application of Geographic Information Systems (GIS) mapping is supported as a means to identify strengths and opportunities for improvement in public child welfare. New Hampshire's foster care system is used as a case study to model how mapping can be easily adapted to other regions. The rural nature of the state brings particular challenges for child welfare stakeholders and acts as the catalyst for this exploratory project. The GIS Foster Care Project employs mapping techniques, in conjunction with the state's Division for Children, Youth, and Families (DCYF) data, to graphically explore and assess locations of placements, birth parents, family members, community services, and sources of support associated with New Hampshire's foster care cases. The ability to assess this system of care through geographic coordinates simultaneously brings value to all involved while serving several purposes. For example, mapping provides agency administration with the ability to graphically assess the distribution of foster cases, thus informing decisions around the allocation of staff resources and aiding in the timely placement of youth, with added attention to proximity of their community of origin.

Although all public child welfare agencies face service usage and delivery challenges, those that operate in predominantly rural areas have a unique set of obstacles that are not experienced by their urban counterparts, and challenges that are shared often carry different meanings. For instance, the concept of distance or proximity has a very different meaning in a rural area that may lack public transportation, easily navigable terrain, paved roads, and adequate attention to weather conditions such as sanding, salting, and snowplowing. These contextual variables and easily overlooked attributes of rural areas are well captured and assessed through the mapping techniques discussed in this article. The purpose of this article is to describe and explore how the challenges faced by New Hampshire's predominantly rural child welfare stakeholders can be understood and addressed through the use of GIS. We present this project as an example of such efforts, with the intentions of informing practice in bucolic settings and providing a working model that encourages others to explore similar methods.

GEOGRAPHIC INFORMATION SYSTEMS

To provide a starting point for the mapping methods employed in this project, it is necessary to clarify the term *GIS*. GIS can be understood in various ways, from the standpoint of its purpose, application, and through the manner in which it functions. First, GIS works as a graphic database that utilizes computer hardware, software, and data to create easy to read maps (Wong & Hillier, 2001). GIS has the ability to capture, store, analyze, and display data according to location (Felke, 2006). This is accomplished through geocoding, which is a process of turning addresses into mappable coordinates. GIS functions by simultaneously utilizing multiple layers of information, showing how each of these layers of data interact (Talen & Shah, 2007). From a user's viewpoint, GIS can be a vital tool for managing and analyzing data about the geographic locations of features, as well as their attributes (Wong & Hillier, 2001). The ability of this method to display data, such as locations of particular agencies and individuals within a population, in a map format allows users to easily see distributions, density, and patterns. Although numerous linked data files are responsible for the generation of any singular GIS map, this visual representation is easier to read and understand, and is often more impactful than the statistics they represent. Identifying the strengths and opportunities for improvement of rural child welfare is only useful if the data is understandable, usable, and subsequently impactful.

GIS technology was developed in the 1960s for the purpose of recording land inventory; its use in academic and professional fields developed later (Wier & Robertson, 1998). Although not adequately represented in scholarly journals, GIS has been widely used across social service settings with various applications. The assessment of large scale social programs is its most common use to date (Felke, 2006). Recently, there has been an increase in GIS mapping literature that focuses on the assessment of communities and neighborhoods (Chilenski, 2007; Faruque, Lofton, Doddato, & Mangum, 2003; Freisthler, Lery, & Gruenewald, 2006; Talen & Shah, 2007). Earlier research that examines youth in the context of place has a great deal to offer current understanding of GIS methods as applied to child welfare. Studies of this nature focus on various neighborhood level factors that affect the well-being of children and youth. Although the majority of this research was conducted in urban inner city areas, this study approach is relevant to the evolution of mapping in the social sciences in both rural and urban settings.

Korbin and Coulton (1997) suggested the use of multiple methods to enhance the understanding of neighborhood factors that influence children and families, incorporating aggregate analysis of mapped census data and ethnographic study. Similarly, Furstenberg and Hughes (1997) critiqued the use of census tract data alone; yet they maintained that it is most often the best available approach to better understanding the impact of one's physical environment. They further contended that the addition of data on local resources and institutions such as police, social welfare agencies, and community centers has the ability to strengthen the methods of such research (Furstenberg & Hughes, 1997). According to Duncan and Aber (1997), a combination of Census-based data and youth-specific outcome data is necessary to account for mediating variables such as family and race when accurately estimating neighborhood effects on youth development. Duncan and Aber were able to extract multiple factors for analysis from Census-level data alone and used six different data sets in sum.

These pioneers paved the way to incorporate GIS mapping in social work. When using GIS to understand the challenges faced by child welfare stakeholders, we must use multiple sources of data, include various community resources, and be mindful of mediating and moderating variables. To get a more complete picture of a system of care, Census data should be used to provide richer context and to account for potentially mediating and moderating variables. When incorporating this body of literature, it is important to consider its urban perspective. Neighborhood factors that affect inner-city youth may not be applicable to those who reside in rural areas. Further, the word *neighborhood* may very well not apply or carry little meaning for those in rural areas, alerting researchers to be mindful of language used in assessment measures and in report findings. Similarly, services for youth and families may be tailored for urban settings or individuals of particular races and cultures; these too may not be appropriate for rural populations.

Although the inclusion of community resources in mapping efforts is vital to capturing a complete picture, doing so in rural areas brings its own set of challenges. Resources are often limited in number, farther apart, and difficult to identify as they may consist of informal supports that are not tied to known geographic coordinates. Although we have a good deal of methodological literature to draw upon, GIS research specific to child welfare applications is still in its infancy, with little focus on rural areas. The following literature addresses the intersection of social work, mapping and GIS, and child welfare with attention to applications that inform practice in rural settings.

SOCIAL WORK, MAPPING, AND CHILD WELFARE

The use of mapping is well rooted in social work, dating back to the *Hull House Papers and Maps: A Presentation of Nationalities and Wages in a Congested District of Chicago* (Hull House, 1895). Presented by the residents of Hull House in 1895, this early mapping effort was successful in illustrating problematic social conditions of the time. Since this pioneering endeavor, the use of this method and subsequent GIS technology has been poorly represented within the profession. In contrast, child welfare literature has been able to provide a great deal of insight into the experiences of children and families in care. For example, research indicates that, typically, children in the foster care system have experienced some form of abuse, neglect, or instability within their families. Once youth have entered into the foster care system, many may continue to experience severe stress caused by family separation and disconnection from familiar people and places. Many also face continued abuse. Further, chronic placement disruption has been found to have serious, long-term deleterious effects on foster care youth (Weiner, Leon, & Stiehl, 2011).

Little research focuses on mapping techniques to measure the rates and distribution of child maltreatment or the impact of access to resources necessary for improving foster care outcomes. In addition, mapping methodology has not been fully utilized to understand service accessibility on a client level (Ernst, 2000; Weiner et al., 2011). Mapping has been limited to assessing patterns of entry into foster care.

A recent review of social work research using GIS found great promise for this methodology and its varied applications. GIS has been used to map numerous variables of interest in child welfare such as incidents of child abuse and neglect in relation to neighborhood poverty levels, rates of neglect and sexual abuse in relation to census data indicators, areas in need of services and those rich in assets, and conflicts mediated by staff relative to season, poverty, and vandalism (Hiller, 2007). One study, using address-level child welfare data in GIS to assess distances between birthparents and current placements of their children, found that youth are frequently placed a great distance from their families and communities of origin (Hiller, 2007). Implications of this outcome mirror areas of inquiry in our project, because distance is a particular challenge in rural communities. The ability of GIS to capture distances between stakeholders allows the New Hampshire child welfare system to develop recruitments for new foster families that are geographically targeted to maintain close proximity between birth parents and foster care placements. This can help ensure that children are placed quickly in foster homes that are close to their original communities and schools. Proximity aids in maintaining a level of familiarity and normalcy in children's lives and increases prospects of reunification with birth parents. One of our project's goals is to assess differences in placement distance among youth from rural and urban families. Placement distance is a fundamental consideration in positive outcomes for children and families.

Illustrating the impact of distance, Weiner et al. (2011) conducted a study using a geocoded database of clinical assessments from the Illinois Department of Children and Family Services System of Care. They found that proximity to resources has a great deal of impact on the efficacy of stabilizing placements for youth in foster care. The authors suggested that chronic placement disruption is the most prevalent stressor for youth (Weiner et al., 2011). These findings support the importance of distance in understanding needs of child welfare stakeholders and the usefulness of GIS. Not only does such analysis illustrate the location of existing resources, but it also identifies areas where additional services may be needed to best serve youth and families. Rural communities and child welfare agencies can use mapping of this nature to garner support for satellite offices and resources embedded in existing organizations to better address supply and demand.

GIS has also been used to map and analyze the rates, distribution, and correlation of physical child abuse, neglect, sexual abuse, and demographic characteristics at the neighborhood level. One such study used administrative data from the Montgomery County Department of Health and Human Services in Maryland entered into GIS software to graphically display findings (Ernst, 2000). Ernst found that rates of physical abuse were more highly concentrated in urbanized and rapidly growing areas and extremely rural areas. Although rates of sexual abuse were not high overall, they were found to be higher in rural areas (Ernst, 2000). This study successfully illustrates the utility of GIS in assessing various factors that may present challenges for child welfare agencies. Findings support the use of mapping to reveal public transportation routes, schools, and various other community resources that act as supports to children and families in care (Ernst, 2000). Mapping applications used in this study allow one to understand distance in light of public transportation and school of origin and to see where child maltreatment is occurring. It informs appropriate primary, secondary, and tertiary interventions targeted to type of abuse and geographic region. The overlay of demographic data, such as Census and crime, allows researchers to better understand communities and those who reside within them. Ernst (2000) found high rates of violence and crime in rural areas, which provides essential contextual information that could easily be missed due to assumptions and stereotypes.

Empirical support for the use of GIS across varied applications provides insight into service delivery and usage concerns among foster care stake-holders. The need for such is further supported by a recent analysis of Child and Family Services Reviews (CFSR) which found that 48 states reported significant difficulty conducting termination of parent rights (TPR) proceedings, and 47 states reported difficulty in finding sufficient adoptive homes (Macomber, Scarcella, Zielewski, & Geen, 2004). Illustrating supply and demand concerns, the Urban Institute reported that the increasing numbers of families referred to the child welfare system has put a strain on the ability of agencies to adequately provide services to their clients (Geen & Tumlin, 1999). An increase in clients and a decrease in federal funding place a heavy burden on child welfare systems across the nation. This imbalance has been an impetus for state and local child welfare agencies to change and improve how they serve families, deliver services, and coordinate with each other (Geen & Tumlin, 1999). The strategic use of geographic data brings a multitude of possibilities to streamline and improve service delivery. The Child Welfare League of America (2005) illustrated the need for statewide initiatives to proactively address foster care placement concerns in light of a 2004 lawsuit brought against Washington State's Department of Social and Human Services. This lawsuit, filed on behalf of nearly 3,500 foster children, revealed that more than one-third had been placed in more than eight different homes during their stay in care (Child Welfare League of America). As a result, the State of Washington was required to make changes to their child-placing system. In one positive outcome, the state authorized a pilot project utilizing GIS technology to create a more effective case management system.

The use of mapping appears to be on the horizon in identifying areas of strength and needs among state-wide child welfare systems. Our current GIS Foster Care Project is well positioned to provide usable data to actively address current challenges and proactively predict future needs of those receiving and providing services within New Hampshire's predominantly rural child welfare system. The comprehensive overview of the New Hampshire initiative describes a model that can be easily adapted in other states to use mapping to realize system improvements in rural settings.

NEW HAMPSHIRE'S GIS FOSTER CARE PROJECT

Although many states have used GIS mapping to plan and assess child welfare systems, New Hampshire did not have the necessary resources until the inception of the GIS Foster Care Project in 2010. New Hampshire DCYF constantly strives to improve services and build partnerships to strengthen their knowledge and research to practice philosophy. They are committed to this project, a partnership between the New Hampshire Department of Health and Human Services (DHHS); DCYF; Plymouth State University (PSU) Departments of Social Work; and PSU Department of Social Science, Geography & Environmental Planning Program.

This project was initiated to proactively assess the state's foster care system in light of national and state-level data. Approximately 800,000 children enter the foster care system annually in the United States (Children's Defense Fund, 2011). More than 90% of states report difficulty identifying appropriate adoptive families, resulting in longer stays for children in foster care (Child Welfare League of America, 2005). GIS mapping is among emerging techniques for system improvement, as it has the ability to provide increased specificity of data with easy to understand graphical representations of statewide foster care stakeholders (Potter, 2005). GIS provides users with the capability to explore and address issues of particular importance to rural populations, critical for New Hampshire.

New Hampshire's DCYF constantly seeks opportunities to improve services for children and families and views GIS mapping as a means to maximize benefits for their stakeholders. In 2009, the state had the fourth lowest child maltreatment victimization rate among the 50 states, with 3.2 substantiated unique victims of child maltreatment per 1,000 children younger than age 18, compared to a national average of 9.3 per 1,000 (Kenyon & Paquin, 2010/2011). In addition, both number and proportion of children in out-of-home care as well as rate per 1,000 children under age 18 have been decreasing since 2003 (Annie E. Casey Foundation, 2012). DCYF has partnered in this initiative due to their commitment to innovation and collaboration, available and usable data, and staff expertise.

Goals and Objectives of the GIS Mapping Project

The objectives of this project are closely aligned with those of the Child & Family Services Review (CFSR). CFSR is an assessment of a state's child welfare performance including child protective services, foster care, adoption, family connections and support, and independent living services (Child & Family Services Review, 2009). These shared interests benefit our GIS project, as well as New Hampshire's Continuous Quality Improvement Cycle. The objectives of this project are to:

1. Graphically analyze foster care case and assessment location and distribution statewide
2. Assess staff and resource allocation and those of various foster care system stakeholders
3. Assess foster care placement in relation to child origin variables, including proximity of birth parents, neighborhoods, schools, and other sources of support
4. Assess the role of proximity to child origin variables in relation to foster child: well-being, length of time in care, and rate of reunification with birth parents
5. Identify appropriate foster homes in a timely manner
6. Minimize distance and transportation issues by matching resources to stakeholder location
7. Reduce the number of placements requiring changes in school settings
8. Assess all the items listed above for any differences between rural and urban settings.

Using GIS Mapping in a Rural State

Like all public child welfare agencies, New Hampshire's DCYF collects data on children in care, birth parents, foster parents, referral sources, schools, DCYF District Offices, and other community-based services. The information is collected via the Bridges Information System, a Statewide Automated Child Welfare Information System (SACWIS) operational since 1997. Bridges manages child protection caseworkers' and juvenile justice probation officers' caseloads, provider licensing, and provider claims. It also manages training requirements for the agency. Bridges is derived from Oklahoma KIDS, that state's SACWIS (DeGiso, 2010). This preexisting client level data is used as the basis for GIS mapping.

The GIS Foster Care Project downloads data (including addresses for referrals, removals and placements, and demographic data for children and parents involved with the child welfare system) from Bridges. These data are then reformatted using Microsoft Excel and prepared for geocoding using ArcGIS 10.1 (Environmental Systems Resource Institute [ESRI], 2011). The data provide the locations of foster care placements, birth parents and family members, various resources (community services), and supports (school and neighborhood of origin) to be associated with each foster care case through their geographic coordinates. Populations and their characteristics are described by towns versus cities and by population density. Institutional Review Board approval was received.

Census and crime data, which provide a rich context for client-level foster care information, are easily incorporated into maps. Multiple layers of data from various sources can be used and displayed at one time. The GIS Arc Map 10.1 software measure distance tool allows one to measure distance between two or more points on a map that represent the location of an individual or resource. Distance between address at removal and current placement, proximity of foster care placement to various resources, and whether the child's most current foster care setting is near their birth parent or close relative is assessed (see Figure 1). For example, the map depicted in Figure 1 was generated to assess distance between the location of children in foster care placements and birth parents in regard to the locations of DCYF District Offices. This map shows the disbursement of the 10 District Offices; their exact coordinates are at the centroid of the light blue buffer zone. Distance from District Offices is displayed in four 10-mile interval buffer zones, fewer than 10 miles, 10 to 20 miles, 20 to 30 miles, and 30 to 40 miles.

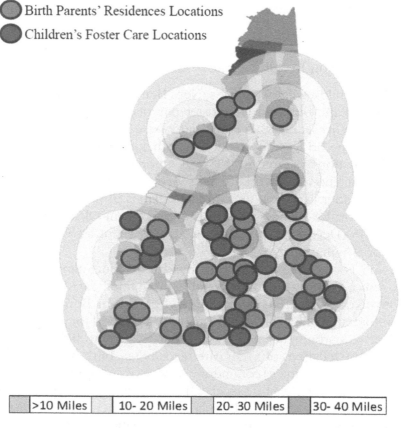

FIGURE 1 Birth parent and foster children placement locations buffered by Division for Children, Youth and Families district office distance. *Note.* To ensure protection of identification, the coordinates of children's foster care placements and birthparents do not represent actual locations. This is intended to act as an example. (color figure available online)

Driving distance between two points is particularly vital as it provides a more complete picture of those seeking services, those providing them, and District Offices. For instance, in a rural setting lacking public transportation and well-maintained roads, a distance of 10 miles may be more difficult to navigate than 10 miles in an urban area. GIS mapping can also bring more accuracy to measuring distance through additional data layers that include land masses and roadways that better depict actual driving distance. Implications based on distance alone are far reaching and elucidate challenges faced by child welfare agencies that operate in predominantly rural areas. For instance, being at greater distance from a DCYF District Office may increase foster parents' difficulties accessing resources for children in care. These findings may garner support to increase funding for community services.

These methods allow us to meet the project's objectives, providing a better understanding of child welfare service usage and delivery. We are able to assess strengths and opportunities for system of care improvement, with particular attention to disparities between urban and rural areas. Further, as challenges in foster care are a moving target, these methods afford us the ability to detect and display trends and potential areas of concern in an easy to understand manner before they become a problem.

DISCUSSION AND RECOMMENDATIONS

The GIS Foster Care Project has the potential to affect policy and improve outcomes for youth and families in New Hampshire and other rural states. This section provides an overview of practice implications on various levels and recommendations for similar initiatives in other rural areas.

GIS mapping has clear benefits for social service organizations and their clients. Mapping provides administrators the ability to make more informed decisions about staff and service allocation based on client location. More specific analysis can reveal client location by specific service need; mapping can identify specific client needs such as a food pantry or counseling center. Organizations that employ mapping are also able to demonstrate specific needs to funders and policy makers. The ability to present data graphically is an effective way to gain support. One can map supply and demand trends, illustrate that services are not duplicated, and reveal how an organization is addressing geographic disparity, of concern in rural areas. For organizations that provide mobile services and home visits, administrators can use GIS mapping to plan travel routes. If an agency requires a staff member to visit several locations in a particular time frame, GIS can calculate the order in which these appointments can be scheduled to minimize staff time and cost while maximizing time with clients.

Understanding what distance means to clients is also a shared benefit of GIS mapping. One can use these methods to assess public transportation, estimate client travel times, and assess spatial relationships between client proximity and no shows, outcome measures, and service needs. The integration of other data sets such as census files can provide client contextual information. For instance, it may be important to know that clients who have the poorest mental health outcomes also reside in areas characterized as rural, farthest away from services, lacking public transportation, and having high rates of unemployment and crime. Perhaps these clients also tend to miss the highest number of counseling appointments. Is it possible that these other factors may impact mental health outcomes?

GIS affords a great deal of flexibility, with endless possibilities. Mapping can be used to assess things beyond the scope of our project, such as health indicators, illness, and disparities; water shed, land masses, and other natural resources; and frequency of hospitals and libraries. One barrier to GIS mapping is the steep learning curve required. Strategic use of geographic data brings a wealth of benefits for clients and organizations alike. GIS mapping fosters innovation; streamlining of evaluation processes; understandable data; flexibility in analysis; adding context to data; early identification of strengths, needs, and trends; proactive planning; implementing system changes based on data; maximizing resources; and improving service delivery, even in times of funding decreases. Incorporating GIS mapping furthers the knowledge base for methods to learn more about social services and adds to the number of scholarly articles regarding GIS use in social service settings.

Recommendations

This final section makes recommendations for those seeking to incorporate GIS techniques in social services settings in the context of collaborative projects. Commitment, flexibility, value, and application to practice operate in a recursive manner and are at the crux of successful mapping projects.

Because the usefulness of GIS mapping may be relatively unknown, seeking support for such innovation may be difficult. Projects of this nature require commitment to rethinking, accommodating change, favoring long term objectives, teambuilding, ongoing program evaluation, reliable data, and community interest and support. Therefore, these qualities should be considered when seeking collaboration and forming partnerships necessary for success and sustainability. GIS initiatives may also face challenges to commitment. The outcomes of any assessment are unpredictable and may depict efforts of social service agencies unfavorably. Because maps are easier to understand than tables of statistics, one may run the risk of increased negative repercussions by using GIS mapping. Mapping data can be misused by oversight bodies, policy makers, funders, communities, and other stakeholders who may call for changes that are not in the best interests of agencies or individuals they serve. To prevent this, problems must be viewed as opportunities for change; taking this stance can be tenuous and requires relationships built on communication, trust, and reciprocity.

Just as there is a great deal of flexibility among mapping applications, the implementation of GIS projects requires adaptability. As maps and related materials are delivered to partners and stakeholders, expansion and evolution of goals should be expected and welcomed. Flexibility may be difficult, testing the commitment of project partners, changing what is valued, and bringing unanticipated practice applications. This brings potential benefits and disadvantages. While flexibility allows for an inductive approach that may be better aligned with real world settings, it may turn project goals into an unmanageable moving target. To appropriately accommodate flexibility, we suggest that GIS mapping projects prioritize goals and recognize limitations from the start. This may be best accomplished by beginning with short-term objectives easily used by project partners. This GIS project tested how to manage flexibility when Child Protection Services and Juvenile Justice Services merged. We expanded the long- term goals to include new colleagues. We were cognizant that this opportunity for collaboration required development over time, and we did not forgo our initial aims for the sake of inclusiveness. Informed flexibility of this nature recognizes stakeholders' ever-changing interests and diversification, while providing an opportunity to enhance existing relationships and build new ones.

Much like garnering commitment from project partners, stakeholders and the community at large may have difficulty finding value in GIS mapping. The value of GIS mapping is easier to perceive when community involvement, opportunities for participation and leadership, collaboration, resource sharing, open communication, and education and training are goals of the project. These components can be supported through project deliverables; maps serve as understandable graphic representations of complicated materials which create community and financial capital. The value can be seen through transparency, project promotion, results, diverse leadership, social marketing strategies, and the promotion of realistic system change. The innovative use of data, applied evaluation methods, and the resulting community benefits, or spillover effects, act as ways to ensure value.

GIS mapping is of specific value to the social work profession. GIS technology provides the profession with the ability to understand the client-in-environment paradigm in the manner pioneered by the Hull House. The implementation of new approaches increases collaboration within the social work profession and fosters new connections with other professions that have similar interests. For instance, social workers may realize future GIS mapping endeavors collaboratively with geographers and environmental scientists to address issues ranging from local to global.

Public child welfare agency goals are fraught with limitations in rural settings. Mapping will aid in improving service delivery and realizing family reunification goals. As findings are applied and routinely inform rural child welfare practice, positive outcomes for youth and families are anticipated. The implementation of similar methods will help others target their primary, secondary, and tertiary efforts to better address the specific needs of their clients.

REFERENCES

Annie E. Casey Foundation. (2012). *KIDS COUNT overall rank* [Data file]. Retrieved from http://datacenter.kidscount.org/data/acrossstates/Rankings.aspx?loct=2&by=a&order=a&ind=137&dtm=10657&tf=35

Child and Family Services Review. (2009, June). *A newsletter for frontline caseworkers and supervisors* (Vol. 1). Retrieved from http://www.ocfs.state.ny.us/main/cfsr/June 2009-CFSR Newsletter.pdf

Child Welfare League of America. (2005). *New technology streamlines case management in Washington State*. Retrieved from http://www.cwla.org/voice/0509briefs.htm

Children's Defense Fund. (2011). *Foster care*. Retrieved from http://cdf.childrensdefense.org/site/PageServer?pagename=How_CDF_Works_Child_Welfare_Foster

Chilenski, S. (2007). Community risks and resources in rural America: What matters? *Dissertation Abstracts International, 68*(1B), 647–910. Retrieved from http://www.plymouth.edu/library/redirect.php?http://search.ebscohost.com/login.aspx?direct=true&db=psyh&AN=2007-99014-123&site=ehost-live

DeGiso, S. (2010). *Child and family services review: Statewide assessment July 2010* [Executive summary]. Concord, NH: Division for Children, Youth and Families, New Hampshire Department of Health and Human Services. Retrieved from http://www.timothyhorrigan.com/documents/Statewideassessment2ndRoundCFSR.pdf

Duncan, G. J., & Aber, J. L. (1997). Neighborhood models and measures. In J. Brooks-Gunn, G. J. Duncan, & J. L. Aber (Eds.), *Neighborhood poverty* (Vol. I, pp. 62–78). New York, NY: Russell Sage Foundation.

Environmental Systems Resource Institute. (2011). ArcMap 10.1 [Computer software]. Redlands, CA: Author.

Ernst, J. S. (2000). Mapping child maltreatment: Looking at neighborhoods in a suburban city. *Child Welfare, 79*(5), 555–572.

Faruque, F. S., Lofton, S. P., Doddato, T. M., & Mangum, C. (2003). Utilizing geographic information systems in community assessment and nursing research. *Journal of Community Health Nursing, 20*(3), 179–191.

Felke, T. P. (2006). Geographic information systems potential uses in social work education and practice. *Journal of Evidence-Based Social Work, 3*(3/4), 103–113. doi: 10.1300/J394v03n0308

Freisthler, B., Lery, B., & Gruenewald, P. J. (2006). Methods and challenges of analyzing spatial data for social work problems: The case of examining child maltreatment geographically. *Social Work Research, 30*(4), 198–210.

Furstenberg, F. F., & Hughes, M. E. (1997). The influence of neighborhoods on children's development: A theoretical perspective and a research agenda. In J. Brooks-Gunn, G. J. Duncan, & J. L. Aber (Eds.), *Neighborhood poverty: Policy implications in studying neighborhoods* (Vol. II, pp. 23–47). New York, NY: Russell Sage Foundation.

Geen, R., & Tumlin, K. C. (1999). *State efforts to remake child welfare: Responses to new challenges and increased scrutiny* (Rep. No. 29). Retrieved from http://www.urban.org/UploadedPDF/occa29.pdf

Hiller, A. (2007). Why social work needs mapping. *Journal of Social Work Education, 43*(2), 205–221.

Hull House. (1895). *Hull House papers and maps: A presentation of nationalities and wages in a congested district of Chicago.* Retrieved from http://homicide.northwestern.edu/pubs/hullhouse/http://homicide.northwestern.edu/

Kenyon, D. A., & Paquin, B. P. (2010/2011). *New Hampshire Kids Count Data Book.* Retrieved from http://www.childrennh.org/web/Kids Count/nh_wholebook.pdf

Korbin, J. E., & Coulton, C. (1997). Understanding the neighborhood context for children and families: Combining epidemiological and ethnographic approaches. In J. Brooks-Gunn, G. J. Duncan, & J. L. Aber (Eds.), *Neighborhood poverty: Policy implications in studying neighborhoods* (Vol. II, pp. 65–79). New York, NY: Russell Sage Foundation.

Macomber, J. E., Scarcella, C. A., Zielewski, E. H., & Geen, R. (2004, November 17). *Foster care adoption in the United States. A state-by-state analysis of barriers & promising approaches.* Retrieved from http://www.aecf.org/upload/publicationfiles/cf3655k640.pdf

Potter, T. (2005). Bringing foster care management into the 21st century with GIS: Groundbreaking approach in Washington State. *ESRIArcNews Magazine.* Retrieved from http://www.esri.com/news/arcnews/fall05articles/bringing-foster.html

Talen, E., & Shah, S. (2007). Neighborhood evaluation using GIS: An exploratory study. *Environment & Behavior, 39*(5), 583–615.

Weiner, D., Leon, S., & Stiehl, M. (2011). Demographic, clinical, and geographic predictors of placement disruption among foster care youth receiving wraparound services. *Journal of Child & Family Studies, 20*(6), 758–770. doi: 10.1007/s10826-011-9469-9

Wier, K. R., & Robertson, J. G. (1998). Teaching geographic information systems for social work applications. *Journal of Social Work Education, 34*(1), 81–96.

Wong, Y.-L. I., & Hillier, A. E. (2001). Evaluating a community-based homelessness prevention program: A geographic information system approach. *Administration in Social Work, 25*(4), 21–45.

Changing Times in Rural America: Food Assistance and Food Insecurity in Food Deserts

SARAH WHITLEY

Department of Sociology, Washington State University,
Pullman, Washington

Poverty and hunger are increasingly significant issues facing the United States. An additional trend, the consolidation in food retail, also contributes to food insecurity. This qualitative study of rural food insecure households investigates how assistance services and retail consolidation affect hunger for households in a changing rural environment. The data shows disparities exist in the amount of food assistance available based on household levels of social integration and social capital, leaving less connected residents experiencing hunger.

In the past 5 years poverty in the United States has increased, in large part due to an economic recession that began in 2007 (National Bureau of Economic Research [NBER], 2010). Although official measures suggest the recession ended in 2009 (NBER, 2010), the consequences of this downturn are still apparent (Bean, 2011). Nichols (2011) found the poverty rate increased from 2008 to 2010 by 1.9% to 15.1%, or approximately 46.2 million Americans. One component of poverty that is increasing is food insecurity, or individuals experiencing hunger (Nord, Andrews, & Carlson, 2009). One result of rising food insecurity is increasing numbers on public assistance caseloads for the Supplemental Nutrition Assistance Program (SNAP); for example, the 2010 SNAP rate use in rural settings increased by 4% to approximately 15% (Bean, 2011). Poverty researchers have also documented that, as

Americans experience economic distress and hunger, people who are poor look to community programs such as food pantries for additional and needed services (Berner, Ozer, & Paynter, 2008; Biggerstaff, Morris, & Nichols-Casebolt, 2002; Daponte, Haviland, & Kandane, 2004; Molnar, Duffy, Claxton, & Bailey, 2001; Nnakwe, 2008). It is important to investigate food insecurity because rising unemployment, poverty rates, and gas and food prices, as well as the consolidation in food retailers, contribute to the increasing issues of hunger (Blanchard & Lyson, 2002, 2006; Hauser, 2011; Kaufman, 1998, 2000; Lyson & Raymer, 2000; Seefeldt, Abner, Bolinger, Xu, & Graham, 2012). Food insecurity and hunger are especially important to research in the rural setting because transportation issues and increasing food prices may affect rural food–insecure Americans significantly differently than their urban or suburban counterparts. The purpose of this study is to provide a glimpse into the food-acquiring challenges of rural food pantry users in a changing rural setting and to better understand challenges low-income residents face when acquiring food in rural food deserts.

Life in rural America has been changing, especially for areas with a focus or former economic focus on agriculture, mining, and logging. Many rural areas are experiencing similar trends of declining job opportunities and populations. Rural America is also experiencing an important demographic change, as the aging population increases. Younger residents frequently leave rural settings after high school, a trend referred to as the rural "brain drain" (Domina, 2006). As many rural areas experienced declining populations, communities also often experienced local businesses closing, such as retail grocery stores (Blanchard & Lyson, 2002, 2006; Kaufman, 1998, 2000; Lyson & Raymer, 2000). Spatial inequality researchers (Lobao & Saenz, 2002; Tickameyer, 2000) have examined the closing of food retailers, describing some areas as "food deserts," or places with no grocery store or only one with a small grocer that carries limited and expensive food items (Bitto, Morton, Oakland, & Sand, 2003; Blanchard & Lyson, 2002, 2006; Blanchard, Irwin, Tolbert, Lyson, & Nucci, 2003; Kaufman, 1998, 2000; Lyson & Raymer, 2000; Morton, Bitto, Oakland, & Sand, 2005; Schafft, Jensen, & Hinrichs, 2009; Whelan, Wrigley, Warm, & Cannings, 2002). Food insecurity is not affected solely by income level of individuals; access to retail grocery stores also contributes to hunger issues.

This study area is located in a rural, inland county in Washington that has a population of approximately 45,000 residents. It consists of 17 incorporated towns and eight unincorporated communities, each with fewer than 100 residents (see Figure 1). The county was experiencing each condition described above. The poverty level was approximately twice the national average; an increasing number of households were experiencing food insecurity and relying on food assistance from SNAP, food pantries, churches and granges, and family and friends. In the past, the economy was dominated by agriculture, but today it is dominated by manufacturing, service sector, and

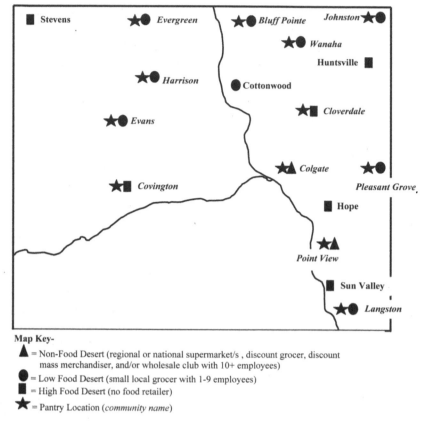

FIGURE 1 Perry County map, pantry locations, and community food desert status.

education industries (U.S. Census Bureau, 2010). Similar to other areas across the United States, this county was also experiencing an increase in gas and food prices, further contributing to increasing food insecurity issues. Twelve of the 17 towns had a once-a-month food pantry funded by local, state, and federal assistance. Many of the towns were experiencing population and job opportunity declines and aging populations. As demographic changes contribute increases in aging populations in rural settings, pantry users in urban and rural settings present specific challenges to communities addressing food insecurity.

The county was also experiencing important changes in grocery retail. Five grocery stores closed between 2006 and 2009, leaving some towns without a grocery store altogether or only a small local grocer, moving some towns into the food desert status (U.S. Census Bureau, 2006, 2009). Towns were divided into one of three food desert statuses (low, high, or nonfood desert). Nonfood desert towns had at least one regional or national supermarket, discount grocer, discount mass merchandiser, or a wholesale club with 10 or more employees (U.S. Census Bureau, 2009). Low-food desert towns had a small local grocer with one to nine employees; high-food desert towns had no food retailing (U.S. Census Bureau, 2009). This study explores how food-insecure households are acquiring food to combat hunger under the changing conditions in the rural setting.

THEORETICAL BACKGROUND

Food Deserts and Spatial Inequality

The rural lifestyle can be quite different from an urban or suburban experience. For instance, population density differences affect the amount and variety of stores and other vital services, such as access to medical care and transportation (Bitto et al., 2003). One trend important to the food insecurity issue to investigate is changes to food retailers. Across the United States, the number of food retail stores is declining; however, the size of stores in terms of square footage and shelving space is increasing (Blanchard & Lyson, 2006; Blanchard et al., 2003; Gereffi & Christian, 2009; Kaufman, 1998, 2000). The result is fewer, although, larger stores in centralized locations (Blanchard & Lyson, 2006; Blanchard et al., 2003; Gereffi & Christian, 2009; Kaufman, 1998, 2000). For rural areas this industry change results in some communities only having access to a small local grocer or no access to any food retailing, or what has been labeled as "food deserts" (Bitto et al., 2003; Blanchard & Lyson, 2006; Schafft et al., 2009; Shaw, 2006).

Food desert researchers investigating other regions, using existing statistics and survey data, found that the food purchasing and health of residents without a store or with a small local grocer was affected (Bitto et al., 2003; Blanchard & Lyson, 2006; Guy & David, 2004; Morton et al., 2005; Schafft et al., 2009; Smith, Butterfass, & Richards, 2009; Wrigley, Warm, Margetts, & Whelan, 2002). Nord et al. (2009) found hunger to be more prevalent in the South and West, yet researchers have limited data on food insecure individuals in the West. Adding to the spatial inequality and food desert literature, this study provides data on people living in the rural West and illuminates the challenges of acquiring food in a rural food desert from residents' perspectives.

Social Integration and Social Capital

Social integration or connections to and involvement with community organizations and leadership are important, not only for food security, but also overall satisfaction with living in a particular community (Brown, Dorius, & Krannich, 2005). One significant difference between living in urban and rural settings is that rural areas have less population density, and as a result community members often know each other and keep close tabs on each other (Sherman, 2009). However, not all community members have the ability to fit into the close rural community relationship, and this affects household food security negatively. Membership in a rural community often develops over time. New members are seldom invited into the community's inner circle initially. Although social integration and social capital are extremely important in the rural setting to combating hunger, the same situation is not the case in urban settings. Food pantries in urban settings generally tend to give out more food than similar rural programs simply because more food donations are available in higher populated locations. For example, in this study area, pantry-using households generally received only one to two grocery bags worth of items each visit and could only visit a pantry once per month. The only other food resource that insecure households could access was public assistance in the form of SNAP, which holds a significant stigma, or through social capital with family and friends or social integration from community organizations.

Social capital is based on the formation of social networks and relationships (Bourdieu & Passerson, 1970/1977). Coleman (1987) defined social capital as the connections between individuals, for example, between family members, and membership in groups, such as church membership or community government, which results in a social network that includes rules of reciprocity and trust. Individuals in communities interact with one another on various levels ranging from familial to civic and along the way form particular social relationships and connections. Social capital theory suggests that social networks have value and that relationships affect the productivity of individuals and communities. Relationships and networks that individuals form serve as a capital because those social ties can be traded for additional resources such as charity and job opportunities (Sherman, 2009). Social capital theorists argue that one of the greatest resources individuals have and can draw on is social relationships (Bourdieu, 1986; Bourdieu & Passerson, 1977; Coleman, 1987, 1988; Coleman & Hoffer, 1987; Granovetter, 1983; Putnam, 2000). This study argues that social capital has a similar capacity to directly affect households' access to food. Social capital is traded for additional food resources from family and friends in the form of extra unprepared items or hot meals, as well as community organizations such as granges and churches in the form of holiday food baskets and hot meals.

METHOD

This study was guided by the research questions, "Who are the people who are food insecure that are using rural food pantries?" "What is food security and access like for people who are food insecure in a changing rural county?" and "What strategies are people who are food insecure utilizing to access food resources?"

Spatial-inequality researchers refer to the case study approach as a place-in-society research design, or evaluating specific research questions from a place perspective and trying to "illuminate the distinct character of" an area (Lobao, Hooks, & Tickamyer, 2007, p. 10). The researcher took a case study approach with the goal of trying to provide in-depth information (Tickamyer, White, Tadlock, & Henderson, 2007) on hunger to further inform researchers and policy on food insecurity. Spatial inequality theorists have suggested the importance of using a spatial perspective to research inequality and moving beyond strictly the city or cross-national levels of data collection and analysis (Lobao & Hooks 2007).

Sample

The researcher decided the best way to learn about food insecurity in the area was to volunteer in pantries to get to know residents using their services. Beginning in July 2010, the researcher attended each pantry distribution and spoke to as many pantry participants as possible. Then, in October 2010 the researcher began talking to pantry participants about the research project, provided each with a study information referral flyer, and scheduled interviews. Purposive sampling was then used to identify households who met the study's inclusion criteria, that pantry users be age 18 or older, be the primary person in the household who did the majority of the shopping and food access, and whose household income did not exceed 185% of the federal poverty level.

For comparison purposes a snowball sample of other community members was also compiled. The snowball sample was created by asking each interview participant if anyone else in town might want to take part in the study. If the respondent said *yes*, the researcher left a study information referral flyer and asked participants to pass the flyer along to whoever might be interested. The comparison group consisted of low-income participants who were not using the food pantries and middle- to upper-income residents. Other than the household income requirement, the same inclusion requirements applied. Pantry volunteers, as well as social service and education personnel, were also interviewed. Interviews were set up at pantry distributions, during volunteer sessions at local public schools, during meetings with county social service personnel, or through snowball sampling requests.

The sample consisted of 65 participants, including community members ranging from recent in-migrants to longtime county residents. Participants were interviewed over a 12-month period from October 2010 to September 2011. The sample includes 30 pantry participants; 9 residents who were low income but not using the food pantries; 8 middle- to upper-income residents; and 18 pantry volunteers who in many cases were also eligible for using the pantries, social service personnel, and county school personnel. Approximately 68% of the study participants were female (44). Forty-six percent (30) of the interviewees were single, 31% (20) were in family structures with children (either single- or dual-parent), and the remaining 23% (15) were couples/families without children. The participants ranged in age from 21 to 82 , with an average age of 50. The majority of the participants (97%) were White, reflecting the racial composition of the county. The remaining 3% reported Native American or Latino/a ethnic classifications. Participants were divided into one of two categories, either a structurally constrained or connected resident. Structurally constrained participants reported not having a choice of living in a food desert, living on a low-fixed income, and only being able to afford housing in the food desert communities. Connected residents, on the other hand, reported free choice of living in a food desert and connections to other community members and organizations.

Data Collection

As previous rural poverty researchers have suggested, sparsely populated rural counties like this county can be difficult to study because residents may be reluctant to discuss personal details with outsiders (Sherman, 2009). Trust was gained with community members after the researcher began volunteering in the communities. The study employed semistructured interviews and observational fieldwork to gain a better understanding of what hunger is like for pantry users in a changing rural county. Combining and triangulating methods in this manner allowed the researcher to hear from the residents about feelings on food security, while allowing the researcher to observe in the communities. Interviews in all but two instances took place in resident's homes; in those instances the interviews took place at a local library and a restaurant.

Qualitative methods in the semistructured interview, case study, and ethnographic tradition were used to address the research questions. The primary strength of the interview tradition is adaptability (Bell, 1987). During an interview a researcher can probe a participant about ideas, responses, motives, and feelings. Probing in this manner would be impossible using a questionnaire or survey. Interviewing also has been shown to be a more suited research method when the aim is to examine sensitive issues, such as poverty or illness, or for issues that have been underrepresented in research (Carey, 2012). Although a household food security survey module exists that quantifies food security status (U.S. Department of Agriculture, 2012), the researcher used pantry use as an indicator of food insecurity. Pantry use was a viable measure of food insecurity, especially when taking into consideration the stigma associated with using such services.

The semistructured interview approach is a combination of preplanned and spontaneous questions. The strength of using the semistructured approach is that unprompted questions allow the researcher to ask new questions based on participant's previous answers and body language (Carey,

2012). The semistructured interviews involved open-ended questions, to provide participants the opportunity to speak about hunger and food insecurity freely in lieu of responding to a list of directive questions. As participants discuss experiences, meaning can be uncovered, which leads to further understanding the social issue of interest. The open-ended questions essentially asked participants to reflect on household history, food security status, food-acquiring and -shopping behaviors and patterns, work life, and feelings about food security issues in the county. The interviews lasted from 60 to 90 minutes. Interviews were digitally recorded for transcription. Field notes were also recorded after each volunteering session or interview and transcribed. Prospective participants were contacted by phone 2 days before an interview was to take place to confirm the interview and directions to the residence.

For triangulation purposes observational data was also collected. The observation technique provides a "detailed description of real-life situations as they really are" (Denscombe, 2007, p. 72). Although interviewing partici-pants can provide information from a personal perspective, the addition of observation allowed the researcher to see from the ground level whether perceptions aligned with reality. The observations proved to be quite impor-tant because they not only shed light on but also contradicted some of the interview information.

Qualitative work, though providing rich, detailed data, is also a complex method to employ because of the difficulty in preserving the anonymity of place and research participants (Sherman, 2009). To address this issue of preserving place and participant anonymity, the researcher took the liberty of using pseudonyms, including altering the name of the county and the names of the communities, businesses, and community members. Utilizing pseudonyms to protect research participants and the study area is a common practice in qualitative research (Carey, 2012; Sherman, 2009). All procedures were reviewed and approved by the Institutional Review Board for the author's university.

Data Analysis

The semistructured open-ended interview approach also informed data anal-ysis. As previously stated, open-ended interview responses often include hidden meanings and themes. Based on this idea, interviews were taped and transcribed for analysis. Once trends and themes were uncovered, codes were created which represented the key findings from the data. Codes that occurred regularly were then assigned as "research themes" (Carey, 2012, p. 218). The interview responses were then analyzed using thematic coding. Similar to the digitally recorded interviews, the researcher also transcribed field notes and coded for themes in the analysis phase. Next, following Aronson's (1994) idea of the stages for thematic analysis, themes and codes were pieced together to create a picture of the collective experience of food insecurity in Perry County.

RESULTS

Effects of Social Integration and Social Capital on Food Security

The question "Are there any food problems in the community that need to be fixed?" provided a great deal of information about hunger in the area. Many of the participants who felt stuck living in a food desert and had few social ties discussed not having access to enough food as a problem. On the other hand, participants who reported extensive social ties and living in the rural food desert setting as a choice reported no food problems. Cindy Shaw, a 56 year old resident of Covington, a high-food desert with low levels of social integration and social capital, stated, "We have real food problems, the main problem is we don't have a grocery store." Cindy feels trapped living in Covington and is unhappy living there. Cindy moved to Covington a year and a half ago when she began living on social security income (SSI) disability; it was the only place Cindy could afford that would accept dogs. Cindy described having to go on SSI disability and moving to Covington as demoralizing and depressing. She reported only having two friends in Covington and little to no contact with family who live elsewhere. When the researcher asked if Cindy goes to church or belongs to any Covington or county organizations, Cindy reported:

> No, I don't attend church or belong to any organizations. I don't really talk to many people. I am embarrassed that I am on disability. I tried to hide it when I first moved here. I told people that I retired early, but now that I get my checks at a particular time of the month and I take my checks into the bank, word got around that I am living on disability.

Besides not having access to a grocery store, Cindy also discussed the amount of food provided at the pantry as a problem, "I just think that the food pantries are limited, that is a big food problem here. For the adult population, people on limited incomes, it's getting harder and harder to make it."

Other pantry users with low social integration and social capital in other food deserts made similar comments concerning the amount of food provided at pantries. Tammy Brooks, a 68-year-old resident of Harrison, a low-food desert, with low social integration and social capital stated,

> The pantry here you get like two cans of vegetables and a box of cereal, two or three cans of stuff, powder milk, rice, beans, and that's it. I would love to have fresh vegetables and fruits, and peanut butter. They used to give cheese that could almost last the whole month. We have gotten eggs maybe once or twice a year, but eggs would help.

Tammy once felt like she had higher social integration and social capital but has felt this diminish over the past 5 years. Tammy explained, "When Bob first passed I got a lot of help from his sister and my friends Dorothy, Betty, and Molly. Molly used to pick me up to go to church then she would drop me back off. Now Betty is the only one left besides me." As Tammy noticed fewer connections to individuals in town, Tammy started worrying more about who to turn to for help. "You don't get much at the pantry here so when I have a doctor's appointment in Point View I also go to that pantry. It's been real different looking out for myself since Bob died, things have changed." The social integration and social capital Tammy had in the past for help and support is no longer available, and this leaves Tammy feeling somewhat food insecure even with access to more than one pantry.

Conversely, food desert pantry users who reported high levels of social integration and social capital did not report any food problems. For example, Ruby Simon, a 74-year-old Harrison resident who has several family members and close friends in the community reported, "Food problems? What kind of food problems would we have? No, everyone watches out for everyone out here." This interpretation by a Harrison community member with high levels of social integration and social capital is in stark contrast to how Tammy Brooks, from the same community, feels about the pantry distribution being limited. The level of social integration and social capital not only affected how food insecure individuals felt; it also affected how satisfied the resident felt about living in a rural food desert. These findings suggest that food availability is embedded within the social landscape of a community.

Participants were also asked, "Would you say that you're satisfied with your diet? Why or why not?" The majority of the study participants who felt structurally constrained to living in a food desert reported dissatisfaction with overall diet, as well as lower levels of social integration and social capital in the community. For example, Kelly Smith, a 52-year-old resident from Huntsville, a high-food desert, reported being a resident in Perry County for less than a year with no family that could help. Kelly moved from Colorado because of employment issues and found the cost of living was cheaper in Perry County. Kelly uses a county pantry because she only had part-time work and was the sole breadwinner of the household. Unlike other residents who reported some social network in the community, Kelly is without familial connections or membership or involvement with county organizations. As a result, Kelly has low social integration and social capital. She reported dissatisfaction with her diet. Kelly complained, "I can't get enough fresh vegetables and fruit." When the researcher asked, "Do you ever receive food through family or friends?" Kelly stated, "No, because we don't have family close by that can help and since we've only been here a couple of months we don't really know anyone in Huntsville." Kelly cannot rely on familial relationships or community social capital to help aid in acquiring what Kelly feels is lacking in her diet, which inevitably leads to dissatisfaction with the living arrangement.

Jenny Rogers, a 47-year-old resident of Johnston, a low-food desert, also reported low levels of social integration and social capital. Jenny moved to Johnston in the summer of 2009 because, "I'm on a fixed income and this place was cheaper than living in Dolver. I don't know if I would say I like Johnston, but it is safer than Dolver and the rent at least is cheaper." Dolver has a population of a little over 200,000 (U.S. Census Bureau, 2010) and is located about 50 miles from Johnston. Jenny cannot drive because of a disability and is generally restricted to buying or acquiring food solely in Johnston. When Jenny was asked, "Are you a part of any community organizations? Do you know many people in town?" she reported, "I don't really know anyone in town besides my neighbor and cashiers in the store. I tend to stick to myself. I don't have family around and I don't go to church or anything." Jenny also reported being dissatisfied with her diet, primarily because of a lack of fruits and vegetables available for purchase at John's Grocery in Johnston or acquired through the pantry. Jenny explained:

> I need more fruits and veggies, especially fresh.
> *Do you ever buy frozen fruits and vegetables?*
> I try to, but they [John's Grocery] don't even have frozen squash and I love squash [laughs]. The last fresh squash I bought ended up being all dried out, I couldn't even enjoy it. I have to eat fresh fast if I get it at all.

Similar to Kelly, Jenny has low social integration and social capital and, as a result, also reported being dissatisfied with diet.

Pantry users in food deserts who had higher levels of social integration and social capital reported being much more satisfied with diets and as a result reported liking residing in the rural food desert. The types of items Jenny and Kelly feel are lacking in their diets happen to be the types of items other county residents with high levels of social integration and social capital gain through connections and relationships. For example, Susan Riggs a 58-year-old resident of Evans, a low-food desert, reported:

> We do have family close [smiles]. My daughter lives in Colgate and my son lives just down the road here [points]. I've lived in Perry County now going on thirty-some years. My husband's lived here his whole life.
> *Would you say that you are satisfied with your diet? And why or why not?*
> Yes, because generally we eat whatever we want and if I can't get a hold of something that we need I can either ask my son or daughter or I can ask friends at church. We've made a lot of friends through the years. It is great having my son and daughter close by because they both garden and I love fresh vegetables. I go to the pantry because I am eligible, but you generally don't get fresh stuff at the pantry. I use the pantry to keep

us stocked up on canned items and stuff like rice and noodles. I used to have a garden every year, but now I am getting to the stage that it is more difficult to keep up with the weeding. My kids know how much I love my veggies and they've started bringing stuff by and then sometimes people will bring extras to church and I'll pick some up.

Gary Buck, a 47-year-old lifelong Cloverdale resident, is a member of the local grange. Due to Gary's longstanding membership in the grange, Gary has built several close relationships and fondly made comments and jokes about close Cloverdale friends. When Gary was asked about diet satisfaction:

I get by just fine. I know this farm don't look like much, but I have a lot of my own animals and I always have a big garden out front. I don't know if you noticed, but I also have several apple and plum trees as you come onto the property, those have been here since I was a kid. They were part of this property before my parents bought it. I don't eat fancy. I've never had to living out here by myself [smiles]. Everyone watches out for each other in Cloverdale. We are all friends at the grange. If I need anything I know I can either ask my sister in town or ask one of my grange friends. Heck I've known some of those people almost my whole life. People will bend over backwards for others that have been part of the community for a long time. When I butcher some of the animals I usually end up trading meat for something else with my sister and others.

Food desert pantry users who happened to be more satisfied with diet were, not surprisingly, mostly longstanding county residents, with average residency of almost 21 years. This finding suggests not only that social integration and social capital takes time to develop in communities, but also that even low-income food desert community members who have developed strong social networks have better chances of being satisfied with diet and being food secure, compared to residents with low levels of social integration and social capital. This finding is significant because it sheds light on different experiences of the food insecure not only from urban to the rural setting, but also between households in the rural setting.

Effects of Social Integration and Social Capital on Residential Satisfaction

At the beginning of each interview respondents were asked about the length of time in the community and likes and dislikes of the area. The decision to live in a rural food desert is a choice for some residents, whereas for others it is a result of structural constraints. Connected residents reported liking that the rural communities were quiet and safe, with open spaces, and a lack of traffic. The two main dislikes participants in this category discussed were having limited entertainment options and having to drive far to get to necessary services. On the other hand, residents who felt that living in a food desert was a result of external constraints tended to be relatively new to the towns (fewer than 3 years), with few if any social connections and networks. For a significant share of the constrained residents, the move to a food desert occurred because they lived on a low-fixed income, primarily from SSI disability and SNAP, and the food desert was the only place with affordable housing. The structurally constrained respondents reported several dislikes, which included lack of community support and transportation, poor quality and variety in small stores, snobbish/very unfriendly people, and feeling very isolated physically and socially.

Kelly Smith does not have any family nearby or community connections, which results in feeling food insecure and vulnerable to experiencing hunger living in a food desert. Kelly reported, "I hate that we can't eat better because we live all the way out here. I know how we eat affects our health, but at the same time we are just trying to get by. I wish we would have never come to this area." Janet Davenport, a 51-year-old new in-migrant to Johnston without any social integration and no social capital or support discussed, "I can't afford to live anywhere else. Living on $698 a month you just can't afford to live anywhere else. It just makes you want to be unseen you know?" Rhonda Jenks, a 47-year-old Covington resident with no social integration and few social ties, reported similar sentiments to Janet:

> Covington is very isolated. I would like to move to Colgate, Point View, or Marshall to cut out the 30-mile drive for shopping, but I can't because I can't afford it since I'm now on disability. If I've got $20 left from my disability, well it's going to take $20 to go into town and back, so what's the point of going to town? Once I get to town I don't have any money because I spent the $20 on gas. It's very, very *heinously* isolating out here. I mean it doesn't look like it is because it's a little town but it's very, very isolating. I really didn't have any friends here until July, so being here alone with no friends [thumbs down sign]. Small town attitudes; if you weren't born and raised here then people don't want anything to do with you. They talk about you and get in your business.

Food desert pantry users who reported high levels of social integration and social capital had a much more pleasant outlook on the rural lifestyle. Shelly Johnson, a long-time resident and pantry volunteer in Covington who also qualifies and uses the pantry distributions, reported,

> I really like helping with the pantry and working in the community. Now I also help with the annual spaghetti feed. I like it here in Covington, everyone is friendly and I feel like I am part of the community. I know some people might not like living out here in the middle of nowhere, but I love looking around and only seeing rolling hills. I have good friends and family, you can't ask for much more.

Carol Dust is in a similar position. Carol is a long-time resident and pantry volunteer in Evans who qualifies for using the pantry. Carol has several family members in or right around Evans and a core group of friends. Carol feels very accepted in Evans and respected as a community member. Carol stated:

> Evans is a good place to live, it is quiet and safe. I have a lot of family right here and I have a couple close friends. I go to the church and get involved with whatever I can. I help with the pantry and really like helping with the holiday gift baskets. Everyone is nice here and we all look out for one another.

The level of satisfaction with living in a food desert that Shelly and Carol discuss makes living in a rural food desert sound like a close-knit, accepting, and idealized rural community atmosphere. Evaluating all the evidence, however, suggests that feelings of residential satisfaction and food security are highly dependent on how socially integrated and how much social capital households have in a community.

DISCUSSION

Pantry users without social integration or social capital were very thankful for any items received at the pantries but also would have liked more food and to incorporate more fresh produce and lean meats into the diet. The current research speaks to the importance of recognizing that populations using pantries vary across and within communities, leading to varying food security needs. It is also important for food program policy to address the community needs for establishing and maintaining pantry locations. Pantry support generally comes from three sources: local, state, and federal. However, population density affects how much funding goes toward food pantries. Because rural areas have a lower population density and smaller numbers using the pantries, funding for food programs is also less than in urban areas. Getting food to rural pantries poses a problem that many urban pantries do not have to take into consideration, which negatively affects the less connected needy community members. A portion of the pantry items in Perry County are federal commodity distributions that have to be transported from the closest metropolis located anywhere from 50 to 75 miles north of the county towns. Transportation costs and the manpower and truck space limit the number of items offered at the rural pantries. In addition, the lack of building space and amenities in the available buildings for establishing pantries in the rural setting also affects how many items can be stored and if any refrigerated items can be provided to pantry participants. The pantries in Perry County are usually held in some form of community building. Some of those buildings had refrigeration, but it was often limited, and the buildings were often used for various activities, and thus the pantries could not store items from month to month. Social service personnel work hard to get the items that are available and to find grant funding to enhance the program, but that is limited to what a small staff can accomplish. How often pantries are open, how much food is provided at any given pantry, and restricted places to store and distribute items are all challenges that are more significant and unique in the rural food pantry setting. Policy and programs should address the various challenges food pantries face in the rural setting, a distinct set of challenges that in the end significantly affects the pantry users and the most vulnerable food insecure individuals in the rural setting: those without significant levels of social integration and social capital. This research contributes to understanding of how social capital works in the rural setting and how this capital affects the level of support for needy residents.

REFERENCES

Aronson, J. (1994). A pragmatic view of thematic analysis. *The Qualitative Report, 2,* 1–3.

Bean, J. A. (2011). Reliance on supplemental nutrition assistance program continued to rise post-recession. *Carsey Institute, 39,* 1–4.

Bell, J. (1987). *Doing your research project.* New York, NY: Open University Press.

Berner, M., Ozer, T., & Paynter, S. (2008). A portrait of hunger, the social safety net, and the working poor. *Policy Studies Journal, 36,* 403–420.

Biggerstaff, M., Morris, P., & Nichols-Casebolt, A. (2002). Living on the edge: Examination of people attending food pantries and soup kitchens. *Social Work, 47,* 267–277.

Bitto, E., Morton, L., Oakland, M., & Sand, M. (2003). Grocery store access patterns in rural food deserts. *Journal for the Study of Food and Society, 6,* 35–48.

Blanchard, T., Irwin, M., Tolbert, C., Lyson, T., & Nucci, A. (2003). Suburban sprawl, regional diffusion, and the fate of small retailers in a large retail environment, 1977–1996. *Sociological Focus, 36,* 313–331.

Blanchard, T., & Lyson, T. (Eds.). (2002). *Proceedings from Measuring Rural Diversity Conference '02: Access to low cost groceries in nonmetropolitan counties: Large retailers and the creation of food deserts.* Mississippi State, MS: Southern Rural Development Center.

Blanchard, T., & Lyson, T. (2006). *Food availability and food deserts in the nonmetropolitan south* (Food Assistance Policy Brief Series No. 12). Mississippi State, MS: Southern Rural Development Center.

Bourdieu, P. (1986). The forms of capital. In J. Richardson (Ed.), *Handbook of theory and research for the sociology of education* (pp. 241–258). New York, NY: Greenwood Press.

Bourdieu, P., & Passerson, J. (1977). *Reproduction in education, society and culture.* Beverly Hills, CA: Sage. (Original work published 1970)

Brown, R. B., Dorius, S. F., & Krannich, R. S. (2005). The-boom-bust-recovery cycle dynamics of change in community satisfaction and social integration in Delta, Utah. *Rural Sociology, 70,* 28–49.

Carey, M. (2012). *Qualitative research skills for social work theory and practice.* Burlington, VT: Ashgate Publishing.

Coleman, J. (1987). *Public and private high schools: The impact of communities.* New York, NY: Basic Books.

Coleman, J. (1988). Social capital in the creation of human capital. *American Journal of Sociology, 94,* 95–120.

Coleman, J., & Hoffer, T. (1987). Schools, families, and communities. In J. Coleman (Ed.), *Public and private high schools: The impact of communities* (pp. 211–244). New York, NY: Basic Books.

Daponte, B. O., Haviland, A., & Kandane, J. B. (2004). To what degree does food assistance help poor households acquire enough food? A joint examination of public and private sources of food assistance. *Journal of Poverty, 8,* 63–87.

Denscombe, M. (2007). *The good research guide for small scale research projects* (3rd ed.). New York, NY: Open University Press.

Domina, T. (2006). Brain drain and brain gain: Rising educational segregation in the U.S. 1940-2000. *City & Community, 5,* 387–407.

Gereffi, G., & Christian, M. (2009). The impacts of Wal-Mart: The rise and consequences of the world's dominant retailer. *Annual Review of Sociology, 35,* 573–591.

Granovetter, M. (1983). The strength of weak ties: A network theory revisited. *Sociological Theory, 1,* 201–233.

Guy, C. M., & David, G. (2004). Measuring physical access to 'healthy foods' in areas of social deprivation: A case study in Cardiff. *International Journal of Consumer Studies, 28,* 222–234.

Hauser, C. (2011, May 13). Rising gas and food prices push U.S. inflation higher. *The New York Times,* p. B3.

Kaufman, P. R. (1998). Rural poor have less access to supermarkets, large grocery stores. *Rural Development Perspectives, 13,* 19–26.

Kaufman, P. R. (2000, August). Consolidation in food retailing: Prospects for consumers and grocery suppliers. *Agricultural Outlook,* 18–22.

Lobao, L., & Hooks, G. (2007). Advancing the sociology of spatial inequality: Spaces, places, and the subnational Scale. In L. Lobao, G. Hooks, & A. R. Tickamyer (Eds.), *The sociology of spatial inequality* (pp. 29–61). Albany, NY: State University of New York Press.

Lobao, L., Hooks, G., & Tickamyer, A. R. (2007). Advancing the sociology of spatial inequality. In L. Lobao, G. Hooks, & A. R. Tickamyer (Eds.), *The sociology of spatial inequality* (pp. 1–25). Albany, NY: State University of New York Press.

Lobao, L., & Saenz, R. (2002). Spatial inequality and diversity as an emerging research area. *Rural Sociology, 67,* 497–511.

Lyson, T., & Raymer, A. (2000). Stalking the wily multinational: Power and control in the U.S. food system. *Agriculture and Human Values, 17,* 199–208.

Molnar, J., Duffy, P., Claxton, L., & Bailey, C. (2001). Private food assistance in a small metropolitan area: Urban resources and rural needs. *Sociology of Social Welfare, 28,* 187–209.

Morton, L. W., Bitto, E., Oakland, M., & Sand, M. (2005). Solving the problems of Iowa food deserts: Food insecurity and civic structure. *Rural Sociology, 70,* 94–112.

National Bureau of Economic Research. (2010). *U.S. business cycle expansions and contradictions* (NBER file://I:\cycles/sept2010.html). Washington, DC: Levy Institute.

Nichols, A. (2011). Poverty in the United States. *Urban Institute Unemployment and Recovery Project*, 1–2. Retrieved from http://www.urban.org/UploadedPDF/412399-Poverty-in-the-United-States.pdf

Nnakwe, N. (2008). Dietary patterns and prevalence of food insecurity among low-income families participating in community food assistance programs in a Midwest town. *Family and Consumer Sciences Research Journal, 36,* 229–242.

Nord, M., Andrews, M., & Carlson, S. (2009). *Household food security in the United States, 2008* (ERR83). Washington, DC: U.S. Department of Agriculture, Economic Research Service.

Putnam, R. (2000). *Bowling alone: The collapse and revival of American community.* New York, NY: Simon & Schuster.

Schafft, K. A., Jensen, E. B., & Hinrichs, C. (2009). Food deserts and overweight schoolchildren: Evidence from Pennsylvania. *Rural Sociology, 74,* 153–177.

Seefeldt, K., Abner, G., Bolinger, J. A., Xu, L., & Graham, J. D. (2012). *At risk America's poor during and after the great recession.* Bloomington, IN: Indiana University, School of Public and Environmental Affairs.

Shaw, H. J. (2006). Food deserts: Towards the development of a classification. *Geografiska Annaler, 88,* 231–247.

Sherman, J. (2009). *Those who work, those who don't: Poverty, morality, and family in rural America.* Minneapolis, MN: University of Minnesota Press.

Smith, C., Butterfass, J., & Richards, R. (2009). Environment influences food access and resulting shopping and dietary behaviors among homeless Minnesotans living in food deserts. *Agricultural Human Values, 27,* 141–161. doi:10.1007/s10460-009-9191-z.

Tickamyer, A. (2000). Space matters spatial inequality in future sociology. *Contemporary Sociology, 29,* 805–813.

Tickamyer, A. R., White, J. A., Tadlock, B. L., & Henderson, D. A. (2007). The spatial politics of public policy: Devolution, development, and welfare reform. In L. Lobao, G. Hooks, & A. R. Tickamyer (Eds.), *The sociology of spatial inequality* (pp. 113–139). Albany, NY: State University of New York Press.

U.S. Census Bureau. (2006). *County business patterns.* Retrieved from http://censtats.census.gov/cgi-bin/zbpnaic/zbpdetl.pl

U.S. Census Bureau. (2009). *County business patterns.* Retrieved from http://censtats.census.gov/cgi-bin/zbpnaic/zbpdetl.pl

U.S. Census Bureau. (2010). *Summary files and FactFinder estimates.* Retrieved from http://factfinder2.census.gov/faces/nav/jsf/pages/index.xhtml

U.S. Department of Agriculture. (2012). *U.S. household food security survey module: Three-stage design, with screeners.* Retrieved from http://www.ers.usda.gov/topics/food-nutrition-assistance/food-security-in-the-us/survey-tools.aspx#household

Whelan, A., Wrigley, N., Warm, D., & Cannings, F. (2002). Life in a 'food desert'. *Urban Studies, 39,* 2083–2400.

Wrigley, N., Warm, D., Margetts, B., & Whelan, A. (2002). Assessing the impact of improved retail access on diet in a 'food desert': A preliminary report. *Urban Studies, 39,* 2061–2082.

Rural Social Service Disparities and Creative Social Work Solutions for Rural Families Across the Life Span

MELINDA L. LEWIS and DIANE L. SCOTT

University of West Florida, Pensacola, Florida

CAROL CALFEE

Santa Rosa County, Florida

The provision of social services in rural areas has historically presented a challenge for social workers. Rural social service disparities are presented in relation to key challenges surrounding the provision of social work services in the rural United States. Barriers that define rurality and hinder the provision of social work to rural families, a multicultural examination of rural community strengths and resiliency, and creative solutions for rural social work delivery are discussed. A case study utilizing collaborative partnerships between rural churches, schools, and community leaders to combat rural homelessness and streamline service delivery for rural families across the life cycle is presented.

Social workers in rural areas have historically provided services through satellite offices, shared agency space, community agencies, and in mobile units to reach populations who would otherwise have no access to needed services. As the U.S. economy has contracted, funding of social services by government and private sources has similarly decreased. For rural communities, this often means that, instead of a reduction in services, the geographical boundaries for the provision of social services increase. This essentially eliminates services because accessing them becomes unfeasible. Rather than accept that this as an inevitable consequence of budget and staffing cuts, it is imperative for social workers to explore creative ways to link limited social service resources with established community institutions like schools and churches.

Resource constraints in a rural community can be either intimidating and frustrating or profoundly motivating. Federal and state governmental agencies and community organizations are forced to take on the challenge of collaboration for the purposes of improved program efficiencies and outcomes without any additional cost. Ideally, when leaders in rural communities start looking for solutions to social issues, they demand innovative, research-based programs and activities that consider the entire life cycle. Rural leaders look for solutions that address problems and concerns while incorporating community strengths and resources.

In uncertain economic times, leaders may explore opportunities to expand delivery of needed social services by utilizing what may be two of the most stable and enduring institutions in many rural communities: local churches and public schools. The unique strengths found in rural communities and factors surrounding the provision of social services in rural settings are explored and presented with a case study utilizing a collaborative approach that incorporates two successful models for the provision of cradle-to-grave social services in northwest Florida. The case study offers a historical overview of joint efforts between a county school district, local social service agencies, and community churches to create centralized service delivery locations and provide sustainable assistance for homeless families.

CHARACTERISTICS OF RURALITY

Of the 308.7 million U.S. residents in 2010, approximately 51 million lived in rural areas (Economic Research Service [ERS], 2012). This reflects a 4.5% increase in population since 2001. According to the U.S. Census Bureau, Urbanized Areas (UAs) contain a population of 50,000 or more and Urban Clusters (UCs) contain populations of 2,500 to 49,999. Rural populations are all populations not counted in either urban definition (Urban Area Criteria for the 2010 Census, 2011).

Rural America is geographically, ethnically, and socioeconomically diverse (Larson & Dearmont, 2002; Lichter & Johnson, 2007). Johnson (2012) explored demographic data and reports increased diversity among rural populations in the first decade of the 21st Century. Similarly, Lichter and Johnson (2007) described regional geographical concentrations of rural poor populations in the U.S., reporting that "the overwhelming majority of high-poverty counties are in nonmetro areas" (p. 344). They found that, though rural poor populations in U.S. Appalachian areas largely comprise individuals from White decent, other U.S. rural poor populations consist of diverse racial and ethnic backgrounds. Lichter and Johnson expounded that,

America's rural pockets of poverty, with the exception of Appalachia, tend to be disproportionately comprised of minorities: Blacks in the rural South, Native American Indians living on reservations in the Dakotas or Southwest, and Hispanics along the Rio Grande Valley and in the border states. (p. 349)

Riebschleger's (2007) rural social work focus group identified "local customs and values, distrust of 'outsiders,' language differences, more traditional gender roles, extended family kinship systems, and a shared experience of stigma associated with the greater social environment" (p. 210) as diverse characteristics found "within and between" rural groups (p. 210). The focus group "portrayed rural people as simultaneously isolated and connected; self-reliant and recipients of mutual aid; and slow to change, while dynamically changing" (p. 212).

RURAL SOCIAL SERVICE BARRIERS

Belanger and Stone (2008) identified availability and accessibility of rural social services as barriers for rural families. Their research compared availability of social services for 15 social services geared toward children, teens, and adults across 75 counties in one state, comprising 18 urban and 57 rural counties. Although limited to one U.S. state, the results indicate a dearth of vital social services among rural counties. Their findings specifically identify distance, lack of available quality child care, and long waiting lists as barriers to needed services for rural families. Similar findings showing an overall lack of resources have been reported in other research conducted in predominately rural U.S. areas (Cochran, Skillman, Rathge, Moore, Johnston, & Lochner, 2002; Gumpert & Saltman, 1999; Pullmann, VanHooser, Hoffman, & Heflinger, 2010).

RURAL COMMUNITY STRENGTHS

Regardless of rural location or ethnic diversity, the unique strengths and qualities found among U.S. rural families, communities, and organizations, such as churches, are profound. Moreover, the resilience demonstrated by poor rural families in the United States has historical significance rooted in family ties, interconnected community networks, and strong rural schools and churches providing needed support in the absence of formal social service delivery systems (Vandergriff-Avery, Anderson, & Brawn, 2004). Larson and Dearmont (2002) described the resilience demonstrated by farm families experiencing difficult circumstances and their capacity to foster positive outcomes for their children in the face of adversity as being critical to the effective practice of social work with children in rural communities. In the absence of formal helping networks, rural communities must work together to ensure that local resident needs are met in response to chronic or emergent circumstances. They must collaboratively address overwhelming adversity utilizing unique and individualized coping strategies not found in urban areas. For example, Riebschleger's (2007) focus group recognized the importance of bartering, collaborative endeavors and "in-kind exchanges among community residents" (p. 210) as established methods of transaction in rural America.

Rural community strengths often include the shared values of self-reliance, importance of family connections, concern for other rural residents, and signifigance of indigenous helpers and informal helping networks where lives intersect on personal, social, and professional levels (Larson & Dearmont, 2002). According to Larson and Dearmont (2002), these strong family connections to the community create a distinguishable social cohesion among rural residents, providing unique opportunities to develop tangible resources through cooperation as needs arise.

Churches and schools are enduring social institutions in America and have opportunities to play pivotal roles in rural communities. In addition to a common belief system and source of spiritual support, churches provide a destination point for families living in remote locations where it is customary to "function relatively autonomously throughout the week" (Larson & Dearmont, p. 824). Likewise, rural schools receive collaborative support from community members in terms of time and money spent improving school conditions, promoting education for their children, participating in school sporting events and activities, and preserving local customs and values (Larson & Dearmont).

SOCIAL WORK SKILLS IN RURAL PRACTICE

The need for competent social workers in rural environments remains a concern for the profession. Recruitment and retention of qualified social workers is a very real barrier to sustaining the provision of rural social services in remote areas (Mackie & Lips, 2010). In the current economic climate, agencies are either cutting back services or disappearing all together. Social work in rural settings requires advanced generalist knowledge and skills to serve clients from birth to old age. Oftentimes, the social worker making contact with a rural family is the only nonmandated social service provider within a specific geographic area and must be prepared to address needs across the life span to link the family to appropriate resources which may be otherwise untapped.

Riebschleger's (2007) focus group participants advocated for the use of generalist social work knowledge and skills and the need to be "flexible, creative, and innovative" in the use of nontraditional methods to effect change. Competence of the local rural culture and customs is key to rural social work practice and Riebschleger's focus group advised rural social workers to "expect poverty and scarce resources; use informal community resources; and adjust to slower community pace or change" (p. 212). A practical understanding of "connections among rural residents, families, groups, organizations, and communities" (p. 207) was also emphasized, while recognizing the interconnectedness between rural social worker as local citizen and highly trained professional. Recommendations included seeking "insider status" (p. 210) to better serve rural clients and to effectively advocate for social justice.

Templeman and Mitchell (2002) highlighted "the inappropriateness and futility of applying urban models of service delivery to rural communities" (p. 767), presenting rural social work focus group recommendations that "legislative leaders be educated about the strengths and assets, as well as the challenges, experienced by rural families and communities" (p. 767). This focus group advised "that the assets of strong informal helping networks, faith-based organizations, and formal institutions should be paired with community leadership to develop information and referral programs" (p. 766) and stressed the importance of having social workers employed in rural schools.

THE PROBLEM OF RURAL HOMELESSNESS

Although rural homelessness is not a new phenomenon, it has received little attention in academic literature (Edwards, Torgerson, & Sattem, 2009; Hilton & Dejong, 2010; Robertson, Harris, Fritz, Noftsinger, & Fischer, 2007). Attempts to investigate the magnitude of the problem in rural America reveal that actual data on rural homelessness remain largely unavailable (Edwards et al., 2009). Moreover, the Department of Housing and Urban Development's (HUD) traditional and seemingly restrictive definition of *homelessness* based on urban definitions may not adequately address the reality of homelessness in rural America. Another confounding factor is the established public perception of homelessness as an urban problem (Robertson et al., 2007). Hilton and DeJong (2010) reported that rural homeless populations do not typically conform to the urban "street person stereotype" (p. 28) of the single adult male, tending instead to blend in with the larger population, making the problem of invisible rural homeless populations even more insidious. Varying definitions of *rural* and *urban homelessness* further contribute to the rural homelessness enigma by excluding eligibility for needed services (Hilton & DeJong, 2010; Robertson et al., 2007).

The McKinney-Vento Homeless Assistance Act of 1987, reauthorized in 2001, addressed the problem of homeless children requiring education by expanding the definition to include "children, youth and families who are sharing the housing of other persons" (McKinney-Vento Education for Homeless Children and Youths Program, 2002, p. 10698) and other forms of temporary shelter. Homeless families with children also benefit from the removal of documentation requirements that the head of household "lacks the resources or support networks, e.g., family, friends, faith-based or other social networks, needed to obtain housing" (Rules and Regulations Amendments to the McKinney-Vento Act, 2011, p. 75996). This updated definition more suitably addresses the circumstances and barriers confronted by homeless families in the current U.S. economy, particularly in the rural sector. Nationally, efforts are underway to develop a more encompassing definition of homelessness to better address the needs of families beyond urban borders and to serve the changing faces of homeless families in the United States.

Rollinson and Pardeck (2006) noted that current social and economic factors create an environment where poor families may be only "an illness, an accident, or a paycheck away" (p. 2) from possibly losing their current living arrangements. With abundant need for services, rural community leaders are forced to develop innovative and creative solutions to address the growing problem of displaced and homeless families in rural America. Hilton and DeJong (2010) advocated that rural communities improve outreach efforts for homeless people and share responsibility for the provision of services on a regional level.

The concept of a service delivery hub (Rollinson & Pardeck, 2006) is a reaction to the fragmented and underdeveloped nature of social service provision for rural homeless populations. The case example is a collaborative "forum through which many people and organizations could participate in serving those who were homeless or nearly homeless" (Rollinson & Pardeck, 2006, p. 39) from one centralized location. Although transitional housing was the primary focus, the hub grew to offer an array of services, including substance abuse interventions, daycare services, medical and dental services, nutrition services, emergency financial aid, counseling services, General Education Diploma (GED) preparation, parenting education, some job skills training, and a shop for household items (pp. 39–40). Social workers, available to provide assistance and mental health services, were located at an adjacent walk-in outreach center for homeless persons with mental illness. As the only regional comprehensive provider of services, the homeless social services hub would naturally become a destination point for needy rural homeless families. Unfortunately, the centralized service concept may thus create an additional economic burden on the surrounding economy as homeless people relocate for services (Rollinson & Pardeck, 2006). As a result, rural community leaders collaborating on creative solutions must decide whether they want a centralized service hub or a generalized service delivery model that serves homeless children in place.

ROLE OF CHURCHES

Hilton and DeJong's (2010) research on coping strategies of homeless adults found that participant interactions with faith-based organizations and local nonprofit agencies were viewed more positively than were interactions with public sector entities. Rural churches and faith-based organizations may take this opportunity to expand their ministries by providing subsistence care and support for struggling and displaced families.

Waltman's (2011) literature review indicates that the need for social services and the provision of service is similar in rural and urban communities. The problems faced by each type of community are the same, and both have more need than resources; but the rural communities have fewer formal resources and must rely more heavily on informal support networks such as churches. Churches frequently play a broad role in providing support and services within the community, similar to that of an extended family. Churches have a buffering effect for families in times of crisis because they provide the spiritual component as well as concrete services to address needs (Vandergriff-Avery et al., 2004). Churches serve as key central gathering places for rural families (Larson & Dearmont, 2002). In rural communities, churches may be one of the few places available to people who need assistance. For example, Boddie (2002) studied 17 congregations in the rural community of Boley, Oklahoma. Boddie found that church members frequently served in other leadership roles within the community or were involved in multiple organizations, increasing their influence and exposure to issues facing rural residents. In Boley, a majority of the 17 churches joined together to form a "ministerial alliance" that allowed them to collectively provide assistance that would not otherwise be possible due to limited resources. In addition to providing assistance that filled gaps in formal social service provision, alliance churches served as distribution points for formal government programs. Even nonchurch members stepped forward to volunteer in helping the community. Boddie noted that overlapping roles in the community among the congregations helped foster the collaboration needed to make the alliance work effectively but also acknowledged that segregation and differences in religious beliefs could sometimes cause conflict. Similarly, the interrelationships and linkages within the rural community where everyone knows one another helped create a sense of unity and a recognition of the "social cost" associated with not meeting the needs of the community. Maintaining a focus on the needs within the community and the overall mission of the ministerial alliance ultimately resulted in partnerships with public sector agencies and businesses.

In addition to differences in beliefs among religious denominations within coalition churches, a second barrier in providing social services may arise when specific religious expectations are placed on families that they feel are unattainable or unrealistic (Vandergriff-Avery et al., 2004). Another barrier may result from changes in church leadership. A change in leadership may make some families, less comfortable in approaching the church for assistance and there is a need to bring new leaders into the coalition and get their buy-in. For other families, however, relying on the church in times of need is viewed as "a source of strength, protection, and recovery" (Vandergriff-Avery et al. 2004, p. 566).

ROLE OF SCHOOLS

In rural communities, schools may frequently go beyond their traditional roles in education to consider the needs of the whole child and the child's family. Gillespie (2009) described the ideal rural family service center as one that is "within the neighborhood, visible, accessible, and inclusive of a wide range of residents" (p. 96). This ideal center would "blur the boundaries between 'client' and 'helper' and between 'clinic,' 'government office,' and 'community'" (Gillespie, p. 96). Research by Cochran et al. (2002) on rural social service opportunities recommends that community partnerships be developed "where schools have consolidated, community service centers" and stresses the importance of involving policymakers "to promote all levels of community support" (p. 847). Similarly, Templeton and Mitchell (2002) suggested that a logical step in the establishment of community-based service programs for rural families is the utilization of facilities found in rural schools. They already serve as established hubs of activity in most rural communities and have the necessary space and trusted relationships that "should be expanded to include family resource and referral centers" (p. 768). Rural schools are ideally suited for such endeavors, as they are typically in central locations frequented by local citizens where there is no stigma associated with entering or leaving and community members of all ages routinely attend school functions at various times throughout the year. Moreover, school-based social service programs need not interfere with the normal school day nor would clients have any interaction with students as they present for services. In addition to protection of school children, privacy and confidentiality would be a two-way concern for community planner. Solutions may include after-hours and weekend community resource programs, taking advantage of underutilized space, or using separate service unit entrances during normal working hours so as not to interfere with regular school routines (Calfee, Wittwer, & Meredith, 1998). Full Service/Community Schools provide social services within school facilities through strong partnerships with the school and local community resources (Coalition for Community Schools, 2012).

SANTA ROSA COUNTY'S COLLABORATIVE APPROACH TO HOMELESSNESS: A CASE STUDY OF CREATIVE AND ENDURING SOLUTIONS

To address the problem of homelessness in Santa Rosa County, two service delivery models were integrated and implemented under the auspices of the Chief Executive Officers (CEO) Roundtable, capitalizing on established relationships between service providers and community leaders, to respond to community needs. The CEO Roundtable is cochaired by the county sheriff and the school superintendent, meets biyearly to identify community needs, and is composed of social service agency leaders, elected officials, religious leaders, and educational institution leaders. This group identified family homelessness as an emerging community problem and directed that a needs assessment be conducted. The comprehensive needs assessment revealed that Santa Rosa County did not have a homeless shelter, public transportation, or resources devoted to assisting with the needs of individuals or families who were homeless. The only identified emergency family shelter was in a more urban neighboring county and tended to remain at full capacity. Other homeless shelters, also in the neighboring county, targeted the stereotypical single homeless male (Hilton & DeJong, 2010; Rollinson & Pardeck, 2006).

The solution resulting from the needs assessment successfully integrated Family Promise, an Interfaith Hospitality Network (IHN) (Family Promise, n.d.) and Full-Service/Community Schools (Calfee et. al., 1998) into comprehensive new resources available to homeless families in rural Santa Rosa County. From inception, these programs used a collaborative,

TABLE 1 Santa Rosa County Timeline of Collaboration

Year	Events
1989	Interagency collaboration begins under leadership of school superintendent.
	First Chief Executive Officer (CEO) Roundtable meeting.
1990	Interagency Project Grant awarded by Florida Department of Education.
	Needs assessment identifies high risk factors.
	Interagency program begins with onsite project manager, social worker, sheriff's deputy, public health RN, mental health and financial counseling services.
	Florida's governor visits first Full Service School.
	State statute entitled Full Service Schools.
1992	State funding appropriated for additional Full Service School facilities.
	CEO Roundtable expands to include local leadership.
	Additional grant funding adds space and technology infrastructure.
1994	Needs assessment indicates large number of homeless children and lack of shelters.
	McKinney-Vento Homeless Education Funds create additional social work positions.
1995	Community recruitment expands to faith-based community to support homeless families through sheltering program.
	State funding legitimizes Full Service School Coordinator position.
1998 – present	Comprehensive policies and procedures established (Calfee, Wittwer, & Meredith, 1998).
	Ongoing assessments target emerging community needs.
	CEO Roundtable ensures continuity of services.
	Federal initiative for Full Service Schools becomes Community in Schools.
	All district schools offer school-based and school-linked services.
	Family Promise establishes longer term support services with permanency planning linkages in place.

interagency approach to secure federal, state, private, and public funding, as well as resources from the congregations and community. Both programs worked at streamlining access while minimizing duplication of services using ongoing individualized needs assessments. Table 1 provides a timeline of ongoing interagency collaboration in Santa Rosa County.

Despite a lack of many other resources, as may be true in other rural communities, in Santa Rosa County there appears to be a disproportionate number of churches and an apparent competition to have the largest number of church members and build the largest structure. During the day, these church facilities are seldom fully utilized. Interfaith Hospitality Networks help homeless families by utilizing these vast community spaces and bringing the faith community together to build a foundation for churches to demonstrate collaboration and leadership in rural communities for about a third of the cost of traditional shelters for homeless families (Family Promise, n.d.).

Used alone, the IHN model brings the faith community, area resources, and schools together to meet the needs of homeless families (Family Promise, n.d.). It is a replicable model with a national outcome indicating that nearly 80% of the families served go on to long-term housing. The IHN also plays a critical role for families in crisis through provision of resources, information, and as a community referral source (Family Promise, n.d.). One of the most valuable services that the IHN can provide is to develop a community resource guide and post the information on a website.

The five key components of the IHN are the hosting churches, day center, volunteers, community resources, and transportation (Family Promise, n.d.). Social workers play a primary role in running the day centers, coordinating volunteers, assessing needs, and providing services to homeless families. It was critical in Santa Rosa County that the CEO Roundtable included one prominent pastor who proved invaluable in bringing in the needed 10 to 13 host congregations (Family Promise, n.d.). He helped to overcome barriers between religious denominations and to get buy-in from church leaders who held stereotypical views of homeless persons that prevented some congregations from wanting to serve this population. This is important because in the IHN model, each host congregation provides lodging, three meals daily, and a variety of activities for each family. Depending on the number of churches recruited into the network, most host 15 to 20 individuals at any given time. Churches without adequate facilities can participate by becoming "support" congregations providing volunteers, food, and expertise based upon individual family needs.

Within the IHN, homeless clients are served out of a central location called a Day Center where clients can shower, do laundry, access the Internet, update resumes and apply for jobs, and maintain a permanent mailing address (Family Promise, n.d.). In Santa Rosa County, the Day Center was first located in a church-donated house centrally located in the county. In early stages, the school board donated a portable unit where the social work coordinator was based.

The success of the Santa Rosa County program is dependent upon an exceptionally trained social worker who serves as program coordinator selected by the Board of Directors based on leadership abilities and knowledge of community resources. In addition to volunteer coordination, the social worker provides direct case management services and serves as a referral source for the school system. The Board handles all of the business of the organizations such as developing policies and procedures for the program, planning fund-raising events, identifying ongoing and emergent needs, and evaluating programs. Programs in existence for longer periods usually form committees to support the Board. These committees may include a finance and audit team, board governance, property management, resource development, and strategic communications.

Volunteers are the very "heart" of the program. Without them, there would be no IHN because volunteers provide the services that range from fixing cars, cooking and serving meals, providing activities for the families, staying overnight in the churches with homeless families, transporting clients via IHN van, and offering special talents, such as hairdressing and financial counseling. As previously noted, in rural communities transportation is the greatest barrier to service delivery (Belanger & Stone, 2008; Family Promise, n.d.; Templeman & Mitchell, 2002). The IHN van transports guests between the day center and appointments in the community.

In Santa Rosa County, the IHN model was successfully integrated with the Full-Service/Community School model. By definition, a full-service school integrates educational, medical, and/or social and human services that are beneficial to meeting the needs of children and youth and their families on school grounds or in locations that are easily accessible (Calfee et al., 1998).

> There are a number of national models and local community school initiatives that share a common set of principles: Fostering strong partnerships, sharing accountability for results, setting high expectations, building on the community's strengths, and embracing diversity and innovative solutions. (Coalition for Community Schools, 2012, n.p.)

Every Full-Service/Community School is based on the unique needs of the population served and available community resources (Calfee et al., 1998). A clear indication of a community's acceptance of the Full-Service/Community Schools model is when the school day does not end as the last bell rings. Full-Service/Community Schools provide a whole host of activities before and after school, and even on the weekends. Services are offered across the life cycle, based on the needs of the population: tutoring, free breakfast and dinner, a food program where students take backpacks of food home for days when they are not in attendance at school, health screenings and dental care for low-income families, school-based mental health services, adult education and enrichment classes, monetary assistance programs for assistance with rent and utilities, and an opportunity to sign up for state and federal assistance programs such as Food Stamps, Medicaid, and Medicare. In rural communities, the Full-Service/Community Schools model usually develops as a community antipoverty strategy (Calfee et al., 1998). Schools may be focused on single or multiple indicators, such as poor academics, drug and alcohol abuse, existence of gangs, poor attendance, abuse and neglect, physical and mental health problems, and homelessness. Community and social service agencies are looking for improved costs and efficiencies, improved service utilization and availability, and improvements in the fragile system of care in rural settings.

Combining IHN and Community Schools into one program and the partnerships between community, state and federal agencies, and schools in Santa Rosa County were critical to success in meeting the needs of homeless families. It was paramount to have strong leadership from the top. The leaders from each organization were committed to supporting homeless children and their families. In addition to leadership from top levels in the school and community, the role of coordinators (project leaders and site-based teams) was absolutely crucial to success. The collaborations were also necessary to secure ongoing external grant funding.

IMPLEMENTATION ISSUES

The implementation of a combined IHN and Full-Service/Community approach demands that community leaders acknowledge gaps in the current social service delivery system throughout the life span from "womb to tomb" and the inaccessibility of needed services for many rural families. Joint community, church, and school engagement early in the process set a foundation for sustainability. Similarly, using data-driven planning, evaluation, and decision making following a needs assessment are keys to measuring the impact on homeless individuals and families to improve the program structure. An ongoing challenge in the collaborative program described here is communication. Everyone came to the table carrying their own perspective of how the model should work. Working out communication issues from the very beginning can be facilitated through cross-training individuals and organizations on roles and responsibilities. Another critical communication tool in Santa Rosa County was the existence of one data management system with a common intake/referral form, which increased the ability to provide consistent services and also facilitated the acquisition of funding and grants.

Templeman and Mitchell (2002) emphasized the importance of educating professional and legislative leaders and promoting essential community collaboration to establish trust and mitigate competition. Social workers in this case study play an important role in educating community stakeholders on the benefits of building collaborative partnerships based on the unique and individualized needs of rural families. They subsequently assume leadership roles in the implementation and administration of the program. Social workers can increase community awareness concerning rural barriers to needed services such as transportation concerns, lack of equitable representation in governance for vulnerable populations, critical needs in the provision of mental health and other social services in rural areas, and confidentiality issues involved in provision of social services in a community setting. They also play a primary role in recruiting and retaining volunteers.

As was the case in Santa Rosa County with a predominantly Baptist population, territorial or turf issues may arise among church denominations with particular denominations preferring a mission statement specific to their beliefs or wish to select particular client populations. Religious beliefs must be addressed while the overall mission remains assistance to homeless families utilizing a mutually agreed upon interdenominational mission statement among all participating churches. Addressing turf issues between church denominations from the outset is essential to effectively coordinate services among churches and to promote seamless family transitions from church to church within the coalition. Similarly, a major concern to address from the outset when coordinating services between the congregations is in regards to liability and insurance. Generally, churches that carry insurance are covered under their existing policies, but each church needs to consult individually with their insurance provider (Des Moines Area Interfaith Hospitality Network, 2009).

Likewise, it is imperative to provide education about what it means to provide comprehensive social services within the community school environment (Calfee et al., 1998, pp. 14–17). There must be agreement among school officials and community leaders as to the urgency of need and the legitimacy of the collaboration. Advanced generalist rural social work knowledge and expertise can be tapped to provide essential training for school officials and community stakeholders on the strengths and challenges of local rural families. Teacher engagement in the earliest possible stages of planning also helps to minimize turf issues similar to those found in churches. Teachers need and want an active role in the decisions affecting their students. Once established, qualified social workers work in partnership with teachers and administrators by serving as valuable onsite referral sources. Similarly, social workers develop extensive social service resources, compile and update the all-important community resource guides, and coordinate essential social services delivery for rural clients.

CONCLUSION

The downturn in the U.S. economy brought with it reductions in traditional funding sources for rural social service programs. Social services once provided through rural community agencies or satellite field offices have been reduced, relocated, or disappeared from rural locations all together. Contrary to the popular belief that there are no resources in rural communities, opportunities abound that incorporate collaborative interagency and faith-based strategies for social services provision to address the needs of rural children and their families. Two such innovative social service programs, which incorporate the strongest, most stable and enduring rural resources, community schools and churches, were described. These programs bridge conceptual ideas on rural social services provision across the life cycle by exhibiting sound assessment, evaluation and data-driven strategies to effectively implement sustainable social services in rural communities.

REFERENCES

Belanger, K., & Stone, W. (2008). The social service divide: Service availability in rural versus urban counties and impact on child welfare outcomes. *Child Welfare, 87*(4), 101–124.

Blank, M. J., Melaville, A., & Shah, B. P. (2003). *Making the difference: Research and practice in community schools.* Retrieved from Coalition for Community Schools at the Institute for Educational Leadership website: http://www.communityschools.org/assets/1/page/ccsfullreport.pdf

Boddie, S. C. (2002). Fruitful partnerships in a rural African-American community. Important lessons for faith-based initiatives. *Journal of Applied Behavioral Science, 38*(3), 317–333. doi:10.1177/0021886302038003004

Calfee, C., Wittwer, F., & Meredith, M. (1998). *Building a full-service school. A step-by-step guide.* San Francisco, CA: Jossey-Bass.

Coalition for Community Schools at the Institute for Educational Leadership. (2012). *Overview.* Washington, DC: Institute for Educational Leadership. Retrieved from http://www.communityschools.org/about/overview.aspx

Cochran, C., Skillman, G. D., Rathge, R. W., Moore, K., Johnston, J., & Lochner, A. (2002). A rural road: Exploring opportunities, networks, services, and supports that affect rural families. *Child Welfare, 81*(5), 837–848.

Des Moines Area Interfaith Hospitality Network. (2009). *Role of host congregations: Frequently asked questions about hosting.* Retrieved from http://www.dmihn.org/about-us/hostrole.html

Economic Research Services. (February, 2012). *Briefing rooms: Measuring rurality: What is rural?* Retrieved from http://www.ers.usda.gov/Briefing/Rurality

Edwards, M. E., Torgerson, M., & Sattem, J. (2009). Paradoxes of providing rural social services: The case of homeless youth. *Rural Sociology, 74*(3), 330–355.

Family Promise. (n.d.). *Family Promise. How it works.* Retrieved from http://www.familypromise.org/ihn-how-it-works

Gillespie, J. L. (2009). Family centers in rural communities: Lessons for policy, planning and practice. *Families in Society: The Journal of Contemporary Social Services, 90*(1), 96–102. doi:10.1606/1044-3894.3850

Gumpert, J., & Saltman, J. E. (1999). Social group work practice in rural areas: The practitioners speak. *Social Work with Groups, 21*(3), 19–34.

Hilton, T., & DeJong, C. (2010). Homeless in God's country: Coping strategies and felt experiences of the rural homeless. *Journal of Ethnographic & Qualitative Research, 5*(1), 12–30.

Johnson, K. (2012). Rural demographic change in the new century: Slower growth, increased diversity. *Reports on rural America, 44*, 1–11. Retrieved from http://www.carseyinstitute.unh.edu/publications/IB-Johnson-Rural-Demographic-Trends.pdf

Larson, N. C., & Dearmont, M. (2002). Strengths of farming communities in fostering resilience in children. *Child Welfare, 81*(5), 821–835.

Lichter, D. T., & Johnson, K. M. (2007). The changing spatial concentration of America's rural poor population. *Rural Sociology, 72*(3), 331–358.

Mackie, P. F., & Lips, R. A. (2010). Is there really a problem with hiring rural social service staff? An exploratory study among social service supervisors in rural Minnesota. *Families in Society: The Journal of Contemporary Social Services, 91*(4), 433–439. doi:10.1606/1044-3894.4035

McKinney-Vento Education for Homeless Children and Youths Program. (2002, March 8). *Federal Register, 67*(47), 10698. Retrieved from http://www2.ed.gov/legislation/FedRegister/other/2002-1/030802a.html

Pullmann, M. D., VanHooser, S., Hoffman, C., & Heflinger, C. A. (2010). Barriers to and supports of family participation in a rural system of care for children with serious emotional problems. *Community Mental Health Journal, 46*, 211–220. doi:10.1007/s10597-009-9208-5

Riebschleger, J. (2007). Social workers' suggestions for effective rural practice. *Families in Society: The Journal of Contemporary Social Services, 88*(2), 203–4213. doi:10.1606/1044-3894.3618

Robertson, M., Harris, N., Fritz, N., Noftsinger, R., & Fischer, P. (2007, March). Symposium conducted for the National Symposium on Homelessness Research, Washington, DC.

Rollinson, P. A., & Pardeck, J. T. (2006). *Homelessness in rural America: Policy and practice.* New York, NY: Hawthorne Press.

Rules and Regulations Amendments to the McKinney-Vento Act. (2011, December 5). *Federal Register, 76*(233), 75996.

Templeman, S. B., & Mitchell, L. (2002). Challenging the one-size-fits-all myth: Findings and solutions from a statewide focus group of rural social workers. *Child Welfare, 81*(5), 757–772.

Urban Area Criteria for the 2010 Census; Notice. (2011, August 24). *Federal Register, 76*(164), 53043. Retrieved from http://www.census.gov/geo/www/ua/fedregv7n164.pdf

Vandergriff-Avery, M., Anderson, E. A., & Braun, B. (2004). Resiliency capacities among rural low-income families. *Families in Society: The Journal of Contemporary Social Services, 85*, 562–570.

Waltman, G. H. (2011). Reflections on rural social work. *Families in Society: The Journal of Contemporary Social Services, 92*(2), 236–239. doi:10.1606/1044-3894.1091

A Participant-Informed Model for Preventing Teen Pregnancy in a Rural Latino Community

YVETTE MURPHY-ERBY, KIMBERLY STAUSS, and
EDWAR F. ESTUPINIAN

School of Social Work, University of Arkansas, Fayetteville, Arkansas

Recognizing the need for health prevention efforts that are tailored to the needs of Latinos in rural communities, the researchers utilized focus groups to ascertain the perspectives of Latino children and their parents who participated in a teen pregnancy prevention program. This article presents a Latino-driven conceptual design of an evidence-informed comprehensive, community-based, and culturally sensitive teen-pregnancy prevention program. The new model, called the Family-Festival Prevention Model, (1) used culturally relevant and experiential learning activities, (2) promoted community connections, (3) incorporated strategies that engaged fathers, and (4) engaged important faith-based and community stakeholders to involve the whole community in prevention efforts.

The relationship between teen pregnancy and numerous adverse indicators of health and well-being have been widely studied and are clearly understood (Abma, Martinez, Mosher, & Dawson, 2004; Hallfors et al., 2004; Holcombe, Manlove, & Ikramullah, 2008). Consequently, over the past few years a multitude of federal and philanthropic resources have supported widespread dissemination or "taking to scale" evidence-based interventions and practices (Grantmakers for Effective Organizations, 2011). For several years the emergent promising and evidence-based models have been noted for reducing the teen pregnancy rate; preventing teen pregnancy is one of the Center for Disease

Control's (CDC; 2011) six public health priorities and a part of President Obama's Teen Pregnancy Prevention Initiative. Nonetheless, teen pregnancy remains a major problem, more so in the United States than in other developed countries at an estimated cost of $9 billion a year in taxpayer dollars (CDC, 2011).

In the United States, another element of concern is the ongoing disparity between rates of pregnancy by ethnicity and location (Guttmacher Institute, 2010). For example, the rate of teen pregnancy for Latina teens is double that of their White, non-Hispanic counterparts in some parts of the country (CDC, 2011) and southern states typically have higher birth rates than northern states (Guttmacher Institute, 2010). Furthermore, albeit the overall teen pregnancy rate decreased by about 37% between 1991 and 2009, such decline was not evident for Latinas (CDC, 2011). During the same time frame, the teen pregnancy rates only decreased by 33% for Latinas, a much lower decrease compared to non-Hispanic Whites (41%) and African Americans (50%) (CDC, 2011). In regards to location, the top 10 states with the highest rates of teen pregnancy were all in the South except for Delaware, which was ranked sixth (Guttmacher Institute, 2010).

These stark disparities highlight the need for a greater consideration of the contextual issues that may be unique to rural, southern, and Latino communities. The significance of considering intersecting social inequalities such as race, class, and gender in the lives and experiences of marginalized populations is highlighted in the literature (Collins, 1993; Norris, Zajicek, Murphy-Erby, 2010; Weber, 2006; Wells, 2002). Additionally, one's social location is increasingly highlighted in the literature as a significant determinant of health outcomes and health status, and a contributing factor to growing health disparities (Marmot, 2005). Yet few studies have attempted to understand the intersecting factors within these communities, particularly as it relates to teenage sexual health (Guilamo-Ramos, Bouris, Jaccard, Lesesne, & Ballan, 2009). There are very few promising or evidence-based teen pregnancy prevention models based on theoretical frameworks that specifically and intentionally consider the social, cultural, or historical location of Latino youths and families (Murphy, Stauss, Boyas, & Bivens, 2011), the rural communities in which they live (Blinn-Pike, 2008), or the values to which they ascribe. Some attribute the overrepresentation of Latinas in the teen pregnancy rate to the lack of interventions that consider the social, cultural, and historical experiences of the Latino population (Wilkinson-Lee & Russell, 2006). To address this disparity, the aim of this article is to highlight the need for and to present the design of an evidence-informed comprehensive, community-based, and culturally sensitive teen-pregnancy prevention program conceptualized by and for a rural Latino community. To provide a foundation for understanding, we present current research regarding teen pregnancy, the theoretical underpinnings of our model, and an overview of how it was developed. We conclude with an overview of the preplanning process, the intervention day, and implications for future research.

LITERATURE REVIEW

Many teen pregnancy prevention programs are experiencing success, but there continues to be a disparity in regards to teen pregnancy prevention efforts in rural areas and those that target Latino(a) youth. When looking specifically at these two intersecting factors, the state of Arkansas is highlighted in this project. According to the U.S. Census Bureau (2010), Arkansas's 2010 population was estimated to be 2,937,979; the state currently ranks fourth in the United States for the number of people in poverty and in teen pregnancy rates (Kaiser Foundation, 2011). Arkansas's rural communities also share similar social and economic challenges that many rural counties in the United States face. Some Arkansas rural counties have an estimated poverty rate that exceeds 25%, which is much greater than the urban areas of the state. Teen pregnancy rates for Latinos in this state are almost double that of White, non-Hispanic teens and triple the rate in some counties, more specifically in rural communities (CDC, 2011). Teen pregnancy prevention among Latinos living in Arkansas is challenged by rapid growth of Latinos in rural Arkansas, lack of health prevention and treatment resources in rural Arkansas (University of Arkansas Division of Agriculture [UADA], 2011), and limited culturally sensitive programs designed to meet the needs of Latino community.

It is important to understand the difference that cultural values, education levels, and lack of resources among target populations can have on the outcomes of health prevention programs. Unfortunately, teen pregnancy prevention programs designed specifically for Latino youth typically only offer a traditional evidence-based curriculum translated in Spanish, neglecting to incorporate enhancements that consider the contextual and cultural factors of the Latino youth, and their families and communities (CDC, 2008). Furthermore, a national review of evidence-based programs by Advocates for Youth (2008) found only four teen pregnancy, HIV or sexually transmitted infection prevention programs that are specifically designed for Latino(a) youth. In addition, considering the importance of parent–child communication, civic engagement, and higher educational attainment in teenage sexual health, attitudes, and beliefs (Andrulis & Brach, 2007), stronger efforts to incorporate these components within the context of historical, gender and familial norms relative to the Latina(o) population are also needed (Stauss, Murphy-Erby, Boyas, & Bivens, 2011). Developing culturally relevant programs and evaluating programs from a culturally relevant standpoint require more than translating the programs and evaluation instruments into another language. For example, Scheurich and Young (1997) talked about the implications related to epistemological realities such as racism and posit the importance of considering such factors in how one collects and makes sense of the data about marginalized populations. Such consideration should also focus on efforts to design programs and interventions that target marginalized populations.

THEORETICAL UNDERPINNINGS: THE FAMILY
FESTIVAL MODEL

The family festival prevention model (FFPM) highlighted here is grounded in an overarching or guiding perspective known as multisystems life course (MSLC; Murphy-Erby, McMullian, Stauss, & Schriver, 2010), and traditional theories of health behavior, and values relative to the Latino culture. The MSLC perspective provides a lens through which practitioners can think about the individuals and families they work with in a way that recognizes the complexity of the individuals' and families' experiences while also honoring the uniqueness of and outcomes associated with those experiences. The theories of health behavior add concrete direction and guidance for selecting interventions for changing health behaviors, and the inclusion of Latino cultural values enhances the cultural relevancy of the model and theoretically grounds the participants' suggestion as to what type of model would work best for them.

Multisystems Life Course Perspective

A MSLC perspective (Murphy-Erby et al., 2010) is composed of four widely recognized theories that together form a framework suitable for thinking of human organisms that are ever evolving, complex, and similar yet unique. From systems and ecological theory (Bronfenbrenner, 1989; Germain Gitterman, 1981), MSLC emphasizes the interrelatedness of the various systems and system levels (e.g., micro, mezzo, and macro) that influence the lives of individuals and families. The context that is shaped and the process that occurs over time between these various systems are significant. From life course theory (Elder, 1995), MSLC emphasizes the dynamic and complex nature of developing systems along with systems' bio, psycho, social, cultural, political, and historical experiences, and how these experiences shape trajectories over time. The theory of symbolic interactionism (Blumer, 1969) recognizes the importance of the meanings that those and families associate with their various experiences and the central and salient roles they assume or that are ascribed to them throughout life. Additionally, MSLC incorporates theories of social change that include the idea of advocacy and social justice targeted toward issues of oppression and injustice as important components.

Theories of Health Behavior

Theories of health behavior (THB) consider the individual and environmental or psychosocial factors that influence behavior change, position these psychosocial factors as antecedents to behavior change, and suggest that though the provision of knowledge or information is helpful, it alone is not sufficient to bring about changes in risky health behaviors (Glanz, 1997).

These theories suggest that the development of core competencies or skills is a necessary prerequisite to bringing about changes in risky health behaviors. The health belief model (Becker, 1974), a model of individual health behavior, posits that key variables of susceptibility, severity, benefits, and barriers are antecedents to behavior and influence the likelihood of an individual taking recommended preventive health action. Additionally, the health beliefs model suggests that a person must be capable of initiating change for change to happen. Therefore, it is essential that preventative health efforts seek to develop the individual characteristics such as social competence that provide a foundation for making healthy decisions and taking action. The evidence-based curriculum Choosing the Best (Weed & Anderson, 2005) provided the content and experiential learning activities for the FFPM. The FFPM provides participants with the opportunity to explore and or consider the susceptibility of negative consequences associated with risky behavior, the benefits of making healthy choices, the barriers they may encounter to making healthy choices, and the individual skills needed to take action and make healthy decisions.

Cultural Values

Culture and cultural values have proven to be important factors that affect the meaning individuals place on talking about teen sex and pregnancy (Faulkner, 2003; Murphy et al., 2011). It is also important to understand that Latino populations living in the United States have different traditions, cultures, and beliefs from each other. Difference is often seen between the rural and urban Latino populations, as well as within and between the various Latino heritages. For this article, research focuses on those Latino/as with a Mexican heritage. Despite the diversity among U.S. Latino communities, the literature does make reference to certain common cultural norms that need to be addressed and understood. In most societies in Latin American countries, the roles and behaviors of men and women that exist today are the result of historical and religious experiences that determined the roots of such values as *machismo, familismo*, and *respeto*.

Machismo

Although the concept *machismo* has different connotations and is understood as good and bad, the associated gender roles highly influence the sexual expectations and responsibilities for men and women. For example, according to Jarrett (2009), Latina women tend to obey men or are often submissive to men. Traditional beliefs in regards to machismo tend to enforce supremacy or power over women—expecting that women are solely in charge of areas of the house involving cleaning, childrearing, and cooking (Skogrand, Hatch, & Singh, 2005; Villavicencio, 2008). The consequence of these strict roles has been linked to social problems such as domestic violence, unwanted pregnancy, and delinquency (Jarrett, 2009; Villavicencio, 2008). Latina women are expected to remain virgins until married (Jarrett, 2009), but the opposite is expected of the men (Stauss et al., 2011). As a result, it is important to recognize that the cultural and familial scripts are highly influential in regards to sexual attitudes, beliefs, and communication about sex (Blake, Simkin, Ledsky, Perkins, & Calabrese, 2001; Faulkner, 2003); therefore, it is important to identify and analyze the concept *machismo* in the communities and the individuals with whom we work. Ignoring the importance of gender roles in health programs can possibly alienate certain important members of the community.

Familismo and Respeto

Familismo means for Latino families that the needs of the family are always first before an individuals' need (Rosselló, Bernal, & Rivera-Medina, 2008; Russell-Kibble, 2011). Also, many Latinos living in the United States live with multiple generations under one roof, supporting and helping one another (Manning, 2007; Skogrand et al., 2005). In the ideal of "familismo" each member of a Latino family is loyal, cooperates, cares, relies on, and has a close relationship with his or her family members (Crockett, Brown, Russell, & Shen, 2007; Jarrett, 2009). In addition, all members of a Latino family (uncles, cousins, aunts, etc.) stay close and openly communicate to help each other, either emotionally or economically.

According to cultural studies, "familismo" will not work without "respeto" because "respeto" is the quality that Latinos and Latinas must have when it comes to their family members and those outside their family (Manning, 2007). More importantly, Latinos and Latinas not only respect their nuclear family members (father, mother, etc.), they also must respect their elders (grandfather, grandmother, etc.), and anyone else outside their family who are older than they (Crockett et al., 2007). Respeto is also significant when considering the importance of the family and the community. Behavior that goes against cultural norms brings shame and shows disrespect for the family and community.

Respeto and familismo provide powerful guiding frameworks for Latino families and, when combined, emphasize a collectivistic community as opposed to an individualistic one. The Latino culture (traditional) is considered to be more of a collective culture, members often living together, with strong expectations of respect.

Traditionally, all the family members are socialized toward these cultural values through communication (Guilamo-Ramos et. al., 2006). This family dialogue is also an essential component when understanding the process of parent–child communication about sexual expectations (Stauss et al., 2011). According to Stauss et al. (2011), not only were male and female youth socialized differently in their roles in regards to sex prevention, this juxtaposition inhibited the fathers' participation and the process during these conversations. Several studies have reported that for the Latino family, these conversations are infrequent and almost always involve the mothers without input from the fathers (Murphy-Erby et al., 2011; Stauss et al., 2011). The content is basically biological in nature (El-Shaieb & Wurtele, 2009) or solely on the topic of the consequences of having sex (Guilamo-Ramos et al., 2006). These conversations also usually include only the girls (Stauss et al., 2011). As a result, talking about sex is uncomfortable for the Latino families for various reasons. The violation of these cultural taboos partially explains the difficulty programs have in regards to recruiting rural Latino families in teenage pregnancy prevention programs. Another cultural challenge when trying to involve Latino families is the influence of religion. González-López (2003) reported that Catholicism's strict moral code, focusing on the importance of premarital virginity, strongly influences Latino's attitudes and beliefs about sex. This may be more of a factor for first-generation immigrants or the parents of the youth participants. Murphy-Erby et al.'s (2011) study confirmed that, for Latino, first-generation parents, religion was often their guide to sexual behavior and attitudes. But compared to African Americans and non-Hispanic White youths, Latino youth were least likely to report that religion was the reason they did not have sex (Abma et al., 2004) but that parental and cultural prohibitions were important (Flores, Eyre, & Millstein, 1998). This divergent attitude between first-generation Latinos and their children is another important factor to include when developing such programs. Recognizing the importance of these cultural values, the FFPM paid careful attention to delivering the intervention in a manner that incorporated the concepts of family and respect and also recognized the importance of gender roles.

CONCEPTUAL MODEL

Overview of the Pilot Project

We arrived at this conceptual model while collecting data on a longitudinal study evaluating a rural community-based teen pregnancy prevention program in Mena, Arkansas (located in the Ouachita Mountains of southern Arkansas). The initial multidimensional teen pregnancy prevention program (Stauss, Boyas, & Murphy-Erby, 2012) provided school-based pregnancy prevention curriculum, community-based activities, service learning projects, and parent education opportunities to sixth-grade youths. The program also included a parent component; however, siblings of the identified child participant were not able to participate in the intervention.

While completing a process evaluation during the first year of the project, the researchers reviewed recruitment and retention data and completed one-to-one interviews with participants. The process evaluation highlighted several concerns including that the program was struggling to recruit and retain Latino teens and their parents. Out of 125 teen participants, only 15 of these participants self-identified as Latino. Consequently, the researchers conducted focus groups with the Latino participants to gain their input on the program and possible reasons for low participation and retention rates. Through the focus groups, the researchers gained insight about the participants' perceptions of the impediments to program engagement and their ideas for program enhancements to increase Latino family participation. Although in-depth exploration of impediments to engagement and suggested program enhancements is beyond the intent of this article, it is important to share the basic findings of these interviews; it is from these data that the conceptual model was developed. The full results were presented in a report provided to the program, and an article will be forthcoming. Although a small group, the Latino participants who were involved in the Voice for Health Choices Program had very positive perceptions of the teen pregnancy prevention program they had just completed. As a result of their participation, positive outcomes were realized. However, the parent and youth participants consistently wished there had been greater participation within their Hispanic community, particularly greater involvement of the fathers. These participants suggested that more attention is needed to address issues relative to the social location and social context of the individuals in their community if programs such as these want greater involvement of the Hispanic community.

In regard to engagement challenges, the participants reported several factors that might inhibit someone in their community from participating. First and foremost, they reflected that their cultural scripts and experiences, as well as religious beliefs, were highly influential in program participation. They consistently said that sex communication rarely occurred between Latino parents and children in their community, and they perceived that many in their community were afraid or very uncomfortable discussing sex. Latino participants also confirmed that, because their religion (Catholicism) is so embedded in their culture and teen abstinence is the only message conveyed, participation in such a program provided through the school was considered highly suspect.

This leads to the second and third impediments of participation, which involve miscommunication or misinformation about the program activities and the language barrier. Previous experiences with culturally insensitive programs, communities, and schools had engendered fear and lack of trust within the local Latino community. Consequently, the participants surmised that families from their community did not understand or want to risk participating in a program designed to "talk about sex." They believed that many of the parents thought that if they actually dialogued openly about sex with their teenager, their teenagers would know how to protect themselves and subsequently end up having sex. This fear came, first, from not understanding the goals of the program, and second, from a lack of trust of the dominant community's sensitivity to their community's norms around sexual issues. Previous language barriers and lack of sensitivity to cultural issues resulted in a significant impediment to program participation.

The fourth perceived impediment had to do with the rural context of this community. The participants related that their community was close in many ways, and this closeness could perhaps decrease the desire to participate in a health prevention program, particularly one focused on sex. Due to the possibility of rumors and "it's like everybody's business," the participants said it was hard to let others know they were participating in a pregnancy prevention program.

Finally, the participants discussed the challenge of the time commitment involved in participating in such a program. Even though the focus group participants consistently affirmed the importance of having the fathers there, the fathers' work schedules often interfered with any participation. In this particular community, a large majority of the Latinos work in local chicken facilities, where shifts range all through the day and evenings. The participants stated that many of the men worked long hours, sometimes 6 days a week. Because the program activities were usually scheduled during the afternoons or evenings, the fathers were either working or resting for another late shift.

Presentation of the Conceptual Model

Generally, evidence-based interventions including teen pregnancy prevention efforts posit three primary or core components: (1) an evidence-informed curriculum, (2) competent and engaged staff who can implement the program with fidelity, and (3) a supportive community- or school-based setting. Although such programs are known to produce positive results, there is a need to tailor traditional efforts by reconceptualizing interventions and placing the needs and experiences of rural Latino/a individuals, families, and communities at the center. Toward this end, we present a conceptual model that focuses on a process grounded in the individual and community experiences of the Latino/a experience. Our model suggests that this process should drive all intervention efforts, including the selection and implementation of the key components, the enhanced content, and the program structure, particularly in rural areas. The members of the community are included in all aspects of the process, from the selection and implementation of the key components to the program structure.

The Latino parents suggested that, for their community, the optimum intervention would include the same content that was delivered through the initial program but enhanced to consider and address cultural and other contextual issues relative to their particular community. In terms of program structure, the participants suggested that interventions should include strategies to engage fathers and involve trusted community stakeholders to help recruit participants and gain community buy-in for the program. In addition, because of limited family and relaxation time, they also suggested the program should include fun and social activities to enhance the participation of the entire Latino family. Along these same lines, the participants were concerned that the original intervention focused only on the target child and suggested that enhanced intervention should take a family-oriented approach and involve all members of the family. Finally, it was determined that the program structure should be grounded in a social change and empowerment-based perspective.

Primary Aims of the Model

Primary aims were developed to summarize feedback and enhanced components.

1. To present a culturally relevant intervention and evaluation by
   a. focusing on the entire family, taking an intergenerational/extended family approach
   b. including family- and community-oriented social events as a key component of the intervention
   c. recognizing the relevance of immigration by providing opportunities and space for the significance of this issue to the community's experience to be discussed and considered
   d. being aware of and respecting cultural values and positions.
2. To ensure the method is grounded in a community-based participatory approach, meaning that the members of the community are engaged in the planning and implementation phases and that their voices and perceptions are included in the evaluation process and in the plans for disseminating the evaluation findings.
3. To ensure that the psychoeducational interventions and activities include experientially based and symbolic learning activities (meanings and symbols).
4. To ensure that the model promotes community connections. Specific suggestions included
   a. incorporating a community festival that would bring together multiple generations, extended family, and community members
   b. including the faith community as a major partner in planning, implementing, and recruiting participants for the program
   c. ensuring that the model incorporates strategies that engage fathers and engages employers in promoting work-place policies and strategies to promote the involvement of parents in prevention efforts.

CORE COMPONENTS

Although the FFPM includes the traditional core components included in most evidence-based prevention models, such as an evidenced-based or evidence-informed curriculum; competent, well-trained, culturally sensitive, and engaged staff; and a supportive community or school-based setting, it differs with regard to the manner in which it emphasizes four constructs: social location and place, content, delivery, and an emphasis on connection and community.

The focus on social location is strategically placed at the center of the model and considers the micro-, mezzo-, and macro social, cultural, and historical experiences (present, past, and future) and the associated meanings that shape the experiences of being Latino and living in a rural community. Additionally, aspects of community- and place-based approaches are essential to educational-type interventions as they provide for increased engagement and clear understanding of the target population's reality by incorporating the group's place, social location, and experiences in the world as salient to the educational intervention or learning process (Gruenewald, 2008; Smith, 2002). In terms of content, the model focuses on cultural issues, the generational messages and myths, and the gendered expectations that shape the Latino experience and influence ideologies, messages, and practices relative to parent–child communication about sex. In terms of delivery, the model includes the suggestions from the participants about the importance of using experientially based activities, symbolic reminders, and strategies to be more inclusive of fathers, the entire family, and faith-based entities. Additionally, from the theoretical framework, the significance of a social change and empowerment perspective and the respect for cultural values was added. Although connection and community were identified by the participants as aspects of a culturally responsive and preferred style of delivery, their significance led to them being included as a separate construct, highlighting connection, community, and socialization and operationalized as a family festival.

Preplanning

According to the focus group participants it was important to include the church and other trusted institutions from the community to spread the word and make the community aware of the program. Several meetings were scheduled months ahead of the festival to instill buy-in, support, and collaboration from these important community entities. Several of the stakeholders were also trained in the activities and curricula so messages and activities could be continued if the community desired. We believe that this initial ground work, including trusted community stakeholders, resulted in greater participation throughout the community. Also, it was particularly important to involve and engage the fathers of this community by scheduling the event on a weekend and including activities that were relaxing and playful.

Overview of the Day

Even though the same curriculum was used throughout the event, some changes were made to help increase the comfort level of the youths and parents. In the morning the parents and youths were separated. The parents were in the main auditorium, whereas the youths were placed into various groups depending on their age. There was a group for youths between ages 9 and 13, a group for youths between ages 14 and 17, and even a group and daycare for the youngest children. The youngest children did not receive any of the curricula but they did participate in various other youth development activities that allowed them to contribute to the family festival. For example, they decorated cupcakes, painted pictures, and made decorations for the family festival. Additionally, many grandparents, aunts, uncles, and others were engaged in cooking meals and setting up props for the event. Although the latter group wasn't engaged directly in the curriculum activities, they were within hearing distance of the parent group's conversations. Consequently, they often injected comments during the discussions. In essence, the entire family was involved with the event in some way. The curriculum presented to the parents was very similar to the experiential activities their children were receiving. The curriculum provided to the parents was presented in Spanish, whereas the curriculum provided to the youths included both a Spanish and English versions. This simultaneous training of parents and youths allowed for a shared knowledge format while respecting the comfort level of the participants. In the afternoon, parents and youths were brought together in the main auditorium. During this time there were activities involving developmental assets, role-playing, and other parent and child communication exercises.

Throughout the day, Latino volunteers prepared snacks and lunch. As the full day of workshops was coming to a close, the program transitioned to the parking lot of the community development center where carnival-like activities (games, prizes, food, and music) took place. Members from the community that had not participated in the broader event attended the carnival event.

The actual event was held at the local Catholic Church's community center. The center was convenient and familiar to the Latino participants, and the event was held on a Saturday, so that all age groups could participate (including daycare for the very young children). The evening ended with a local band and a soccer game. Soccer balls and other symbolic items were handed out throughout the day with the Voices 4 Healthy Choices logo on them, with the hope that taking them home would remind the participants of their day and the knowledge they gained. Another important attribute of the festival was the involvement of more than 10 Spanish speaking interpreter volunteers and church clergy from the community who were available and present throughout the entire event.

In Fall 2010, this new conceptual model was pilot tested after months of planning. The planning for this event included a large number of stakeholders from the community including Healthy Connections staff, a community midwife, church volunteers, and community parents and youths. In collaboration with the local Catholic church and the other community partners, the family festival was held involving more than 400 Hispanic youths and families in DeQueen, Arkansas. As the day progressed, several community members and festival participants participated in interviews about their initial thoughts of the festival. Also, the evaluators conducted 121 pre- and posttests that day with youth participants ages 13 to 17. A month following, focus groups were completed with the festival participants. The article describing the empirical results is forthcoming.

Implications for Future Research

The FFPM is yet to be fully tested for its effectiveness, applicability, and generalizability. It is informed by the participants it aims to target and builds upon an evidence-based curricula that has been studied. This provides credence for anticipation of positive outcomes regarding participant recruitment and engagement, participant knowledge and awareness levels, increases in parent–child communication relative to teen sex, and changes in behaviors and attitudes about teen sex that result in increased teen sexual abstinence. Future research should include replication of the program, first using a pre-experimental, mixed-methods design and efforts to manualize (to more clearly articulate and operationalize the core components of the model). The next level of evaluation should also include a multisite component that will allow the intervention to be delivered in an urban Latino community and a rural Latino community so the results can be compared.

REFERENCES

Abma, J. C., Martinez, G. M., Mosher, W. D., & Dawson, B. S. (2004). Teenagers in the United States: Sexual activity, contraceptive use, and childbearing, 2002. *National Center for Health Statistics. Vital Health Stat, 23*(24),

Advocates for Youth. (2008). *Science and Success: Science-based programs that work to prevent teen pregnancy, HIV and sexually transmitted infections among Hispanics/Latinos*. Washington, DC: Author.

Andrulis, D. P., & Brach, C. (2007). Integrating literacy, culture, and language to improve health care quality for diverse populations. *American Journal of Health Behavior, 31*(1), S122–133.

Becker, M. H. (Ed.). (1974). The health belief model and personal health behavior. *Health Education Monographs, 2,* 32473.

Blake, S. M., Simkin, L., Ledsky, R., Perkins, C., & Calabrese, J. M. (2001). Effects of a parent-child communications intervention on young adolescents' risk for early onset of sexual intercourse. *Family Planning Perspectives, 33*(2), 52–61.

Blinn-Pike, L. (2008). Sex education in rural schools in the United States: Impact of rural educators' community identities. *Sex Education, 8*(1), 77–92.

Blumer, H. (1969). *Symbolic interactionism: Perspective and method.* Englewood Cliffs, NJ: Prentice Hall.

Bronfenbrenner, U. (1989). Ecological systems theory. *Annals of Child Development, 6*, 187–249.

Centers for Disease Control and Prevention. (2008). *Nation's high school students showing overall improvements in health-related behaviors.* Retrieved from htpp://www.cdc.gov/HealthyYouth/yrbs/pdf/yrbs07_press_release.pdf.

Centers for Disease Control and Prevention. (2011). Teen pregnancy: Improving the lives of young people and strengthening communities by reducing teen pregnancy. *At a Glance, 2011.* Retrieved from: http://www.cdc.gov/chronicdisease/resources/publications/aag/teen-preg.htm

Collins, P. H. (1993). Toward a new vision: Race, class, and gender as categories of analysis and connection. *Race, Sex &Class, 1*(1), 25–45.

Crockett, L. J., Brown, J., Russell, S., & Shen, Y. L. (2007). The meaning of good parent-child relationships for Mexican American adolescents. *Journal of Research on Adolescence, 17*(4), 639–667. doi:10.1111/j.1532-7795.2007.00538.x

Elder, G. H. (1995). The life course paradigm: Social change and individual development. In P. Moen, G. H. Elder, & K. Luscher (Eds.) *Examining lives in context: Perspectives on the ecology of human development* (pp. 101–139). Washington, DC: American Psychological Association.

El-Shaieb, M., & Wurtele, S. K. (2009). Parents' plans to discuss sexuality with their young children. *American Journal of Sexuality Education, 4*, 103–115.

Faulkner, S. L. (2003). Good girl or flirt girl: Latinas' definitions of sex and sexual relationships. *Hispanic Journal of Behavioral Sciences, 25*(2), 174–200.

Flores, E., Eyre, S. L., & Millstein, S. G. (1998). Sociocultural beliefs related to sex among Mexican American adolescents. *Hispanic Journal of Behavioral Sciences, 20*(1), 60–82.

Germaine, C., & Gitterman, A. (1981). *The life model of social work practice.* New York, NY: Columbia University Press.

Glanz, K. (1997). *Theory at a glance: A guide for health promotion practice.* Washington, DC: U.S. Department of Health and Human Services.

González-López, G. (2003). De madres a hijas: Gendered lessons on virginity across generations of Mexican immigrant women. In P. Hondagneu-Sotelo (Ed.), *Gender and U.S. immigration: Contemporary trends* (pp. 217–240). Berkeley, CA: University of California Press.

Grantmakers for Effective Organizations. (2011). *Scaling what works: Building the evaluative capacity of grantees training handout.* Little Rock, AR: Cox Creative Center.

Gruenewald, D. A. (2008). The best of both worlds: A critical pedagogy of place. *Environmental Education Research, 14*(3), 308–324.

Guilamo-Ramos, V., Bouris, A., Jaccard, J., Lesesne, C., & Ballan, M. (2009). Familial and cultural influences on sexual risk behaviors among Mexican, Puerto Rican, and Dominican youth. *AIDS Education and Prevention, 21*(5 Suppl), 61–79.

Guilamo-Ramos, V., Dittus, P., Jaccared, J., Goldberh, V., Casillas, E., & Bouris, A. (2006). The content and process of mother-adolescent communication about sex in Latino families. *Social Work Research, 30*(3), 169–181.

Guttmacher Institute. (2010). *U.S. teenage pregnancies, births, and abortions: National and state trends and trends by race and ethnicity.* New York, NY: Author. Retrieved from http://www.guttmacher.org/pubs/USTPtrends.pdf

Hallfors, D., Waller, M. W., Ford, C. A., Halpern, C. T., Brodish, P. H., & Iritani, B. (2004). Adolescent depression and suicide risk: Association with sex and drug behavior. *American Journal of Preventative Medicine, 27*(3), 224–231.

Holcombe, E., & Manlove, J., & Ikramullah, E. (2008). Forced sexual intercourse among young adult women. *Child trends fact sheet* (Publication #2008-30). Washington, DC: Child Trends.

Jarrett, K. (2009). The influences of acculturation, marianismo and ethnic identity on sexual activity among Latina adolescents. *ePublications@Marquette.* Retrieved from http://epublications.marquette.edu/dissertations_mu/93

Kaiser Foundation. (2011). *Fact sheet: Sexual health of adolescents and young adults in the United States.* Retrieved from www.kff.org/womenshealth/3040.cfm

Manning, L. C. (2007). *Diversity within: A parenting measure for immigrant Mexican American mothers.* Retrieved from http://hdfs.missouri.edu/documents/graduate/dissertations_theses/dissertation_manning.pdf

Marmot, M. (2005). The social environment and health. *Clinical Medicine, 5*(3), 244–248.

Murphy, Y., Stauss, K., Boyas, J., & Bivens, V. (2011). Voices of Latino parents and teens: Tailored strategies for parent-child communication related to sex. *Journal of Children and Poverty, 17*(1), 125–138.

Murphy-Erby, Y., McMullian, K., Stauss, K., & Schriver, J. (2010*)*. Multi-systems life course: A new practice perspective and its application in advanced practice with racial and ethnic populations. *Journal of Human Behavior and Social Environment, 20*(5), 672–687.

Norris, A., Zajicek, A., & Murphy-Erby, Y. (2010). Intersectional perspective and rural poverty research: Benefits, challenges, and policy implications. *Journal of Poverty, 14*(1), 55–75.

Rosselló, J., Bernal, G., & Rivera-Medina, C. (2008). Individual and group CBT and IPT for Puerto Rican adolescents with depressive symptoms. *Cultural Diversity and Ethnic Minority Psychology, 14*(3), 234–245. doi:10.1037/1099-9809.14.3.234

Russell-Kibble, A. (2011*)*. *Mexican American parents' perceptions of cultural influences on grieving the death of their child.* Retrieved from: http://www.nursing.arizona.edu/Library/RussellKIbble_Audrey_Practice_Inquiry.pdf

Scheurich, J. J., & Young, M. D. (1997). Coloring epistemologies: Are our research epistemologies racially biased? *Educational Researcher, 26*(4), 4–16.

Skogrand, L., Hatch, D., & Singh, A. (2005). Understanding Latino families, implications for family education. *Family Resources.* Retrieved from http://extension.usu.edu/files/publications/publication/FR_Family_2005-02.pdf

Smith, G. (2002). Place-based education: Learning to be where we are. *Phi Delta Kappan, 83*, 584–594.

Stauss, K., Boyas, J., & Murphy-Erby, Y. (2012). Implementing and evaluating a rural community-based sexual abstinence program: Challenges and solutions. *Sex Education, 12*(1), 47–63.

Stauss, K., Murphy-Erby, Y., Boyas, J., & Bivens, V. (2011). Parent-child communication related to sexual health: The contextual experiences of rural Latino parents and youth. *Advances in Social Work, 12*(2), 181–200.

University of Arkansas Division of Agriculture. (2011). *Rural profile of Arkansas 2011*. Retrieved from http://www.arcommunities.org/econ_dev/economic_profiles/default.htm

U.S. Census Bureau. (2010). *Census 2010 redistricting data: Race, Hispanic or Latino*. Retrieved from http://2010.census.gov/2010census/

Villavicencio, A. L. (2008). Latina adolescents: exploring the dynamics of family experiences, gender role beliefs, and dating relationships. *Counseling Psychology Dissertations*. Retrieved from http://hdl.handle.net/2047/d10018372

Weber, L. (2006). Reconstructing the landscape of health disparities research: Promoting dialogue and collaboration between feminist intersectional and biomedical paradigms. In A. J. Schultz & L. Mullings (Eds.), *Gender, race, class, & health* (pp. 21–59). San Francisco, CA: John Wiley & Sons.

Weed, S., & Anderson, N. (2005). *Evaluation of choosing the best*. Salt Lake City, UT: U.S. Department of Health and Human Services. Retrieved from http://choosingthebest.org/docs/CTB_2005_Research_Study.pdf

Wells, B. (2002). Women's voices: Explaining poverty and plenty in a rural community. *Rural Sociology, 67*2, 234–254.

Wilkinson-Lee, A., & Russell, S. (2006). Practitioners' perspectives on cultural sensitivity in Latina/o teen pregnancy prevention. *Family Relations, 55*, 376–389.

Rural Kinship Caregivers' Perceptions of Child Well-Being: The Use of Attribution Theory

RAMONA W. DENBY and ALLISON BOWMER

School of Social Work, University of Nevada Las Vegas,
Las Vegas, Nevada

Sixty-one rural, southwestern U.S. kinship caregivers were asked about their experiences and how those experiences influence the well-being of the 122 children in their care. They reported high levels of caregiving readiness/capacity and parenting abilities. Attribution theory, the manner in which people associate behavior, is used to interpret the findings and provide a set of practice, programming, and policy recommendations.

According to the 2010 U.S. Census Bureau, approximately 59.5 million people live in rural areas in the United States (U.S. Census Bureau, Geography Division, 2012). The 2007 National Survey of Children's Health estimates that 13.5 million children reside in rural America (U.S. Department of Health and Human Services, Health Resources and Services Administration, 2011). In comparison with children who live in urban areas, the rate of children in kinship foster care arrangements may be higher in rural areas. For instance, the American Community Survey reported that 48% of grandparents in rural

This research was supported by grant funding from the State of Nevada Division of Child and Family Services, the Clark County Department of Family Services (via a demonstration grant from the U.S Children's Bureau Improving Child Welfare Outcomes through Systems of Care), and the New York Community Trust, Silberman Fund Faculty Grant Program.

areas are responsible for their grandchildren, in comparison to nearly 39% of grandparents in urban areas (U.S. Census Bureau, 2006–2010).

Parenting in rural communities is unique in its strengths and challenges. A few of the distinct parenting challenges for families living in rural communities pertain to the geography of the area and the networking abilities of residents. Common complaints associated with rural life include a lack of resources and trained professionals, isolation, and poverty (Kropf & Kolomer, 2004; Lauver, 2010; McGuinness, 2009; Starr, Campbell, & Herrick, 2002). The challenges associated with rural life are often compounded by caregivers' attitudes about their readiness to parent. For instance, rural caregivers' access to resources might be affected by the caregivers' feelings of mistrust (Conklin, 1980; Starr et al., 2002) or whether they doubt their own ability to provide care (Conklin, 1980; Lauver, 2010). Despite the challenges of rearing children in rural communities and the unique needs of caregivers, there is currently limited research regarding the experiences of kinship caregivers in rural areas; thus, the purpose of this study. The authors seek to describe the distinctive needs of rural kinship caregivers in an effort to provide practitioners and policy advocates with strategies for increasing support to the children in their care.

Rural Kinship Caregiving Experiences

Rural kinship caregivers' capacity or readiness to provide support to the children in their care may be related to their own feelings of perceived support. Bullock (2007) found that greater incomes and social support (e.g., family cohesion) influenced grandfathers' satisfaction and readiness to parent. Research by King et al. (2009) found that rural caregivers with limited financial support were less likely to participate in community events, which led to increased feelings of social isolation over time. Moreover, Letiecq, Bailey, and Kurtz (2008) found that rural grandparent caregivers were less likely to report depression if they had ample social support available to them. For kinship caregivers without the support of their families, community participation may provide the social support they need to promote their well-being. For instance, it is common for rural families to report involvement in a spiritual or religious community (Bullock, 2007; Larson & Dearmont, 2002; Myers, Kropf, & Robinson, 2002). Moreover, there is evidence that support groups are helpful in promoting social support, increasing understanding, and alleviating stress in rural kinship caregivers (King et al., 2009). Despite the amount of research reporting the outcomes of children in kinship care, there is currently limited information about how, if at all, caregivers attribute the outcomes of their children's well-being to their own parenting or the circumstances of their environment.

EMPIRICAL FRAMEWORK

Attribution Theory

Attribution theory, in the context of social psychology, refers to a thinking process in which inferences are made to explain the causes of behavior in an attempt to predict future outcomes. The two theorists responsible for the creation of this theory are Gustav Ichheiser (1943) and Fritz Heider (1958). According to Ichheiser (1943), attributions are made in response to individual and collective interpretations about behaviors that are determined by either personal or situational factors. Expanding this premise, Heider (1958) claimed that all actions are determined by personal factors (i.e., internal traits such as one's ability, attitude, or actions) or environmental factors (i.e., external factors beyond one's control). In addition to these concepts, three primary dimensions further explain the causes of behavior: the locus of causality (i.e., whether a cause is attributed to internal or external traits), stability (i.e., whether a cause is considered to be stable/unchanging or unstable/temporary), and controllability (i.e., whether the cause can be controlled through the actions of the individual) (Salkind, 2005; Weiner, 1986). Research suggests that these dimensions are correlated with emotional effects in both the actor and the observer and may be used to predict future outcomes or successes (Salkind, 2005).

As suggested by Ichheiser (1943), when making attributions for why events occur, personal factors tend to be overemphasized in comparison to situational factors. Moreover, once one's impression of a person has been determined, it is difficult to change or challenge that view (Ichheiser, 1943). As proposed by Gilbert (1998), because characteristics are attributed through one's observation of another, the observer is typically unaware of the actor's situational context or environmental constraints; therefore, the observer will ascribe behavior as being defined by internal personality traits. In congruence with this concept, research finds that when observers tell others about another person's situation, they are likely to focus only on internal traits, leaving the people they tell with more extreme opinions about the aforementioned person (Gilovich, 1987). Thus, interactions with other people tend to revolve around impression management in which others may choose to adjust their behavior to the expectations of the roles they have been previously assigned by observers (Ichheiser, 1943).

> What we can do is influenced by what we think we can do, and what we think we can do is influenced by what other people think we can do. Therefore, what we can do is influenced by what other people think we can do. (Heider, 1958, p. 97)

Acknowledging the relevance of attribution and the effect of emotional arousal during social interactions with others, one may suspect that there is a tendency to misinterpret information about oneself and the environment. One such tendency, referred to as the self-serving bias, occurs when people take credit for success, yet attribute negative outcomes to external factors (Miller & Ross, 1975). According to Shepperd, Malone, and Sweeny (2008), the self-serving bias may be influenced by motivating factors relating to self-enhancement and self-presentation, as taking personal credit for positive outcomes may promote feelings of self-worth and could influence how one is perceived by others. Moreover, the self-serving bias might be associated with protecting self-esteem, as Campbell and Sedikides (1999) discovered; when one's self-concept is threatened, it is more likely that the self-serving bias will occur. In this study we explored the extent that rural caregivers reported positive outcomes in regard to the well-being of children in their care and the types of attributions (internal—their own abilities, and external—resource needs) that accounted for the children's condition. It is suggested that because rural communities tend to be smaller and dwellers are more likely to know and engage with their neighbors, kinship caregivers of this population may be especially prone to exhibiting the self-serving bias as a result of the increased importance of impression management in their communities, as poor outcomes in child well-being could be attributed to their own parenting abilities by their peers.

METHOD

Description of the Sample

The sample, 61 rural residents, was primarily female (90%; see Table 1). The respondents' ages ranged from 21 to 84, with a mean age of 53. Less than one half (43%) of respondents were married. The most prevalent ethnicities reported were White (44%) and Native American (37%). Almost two thirds of respondents (64%) earned $20,000 or less. About one half (54%) of the sample indicated employment as their primary income source. One third of respondents had some college, whereas 43% had a high school diploma or General Education Diploma (GED). A majority (61%) of rural caregivers were homeowners. A majority of their children were female (59%; see Table 2). The average age of children in care was 9.0, with a range of 1.5 to 17.0. Many of the rural kinship caregivers (43%) were caring for one of their relative's children. Almost as many (38%) were caring for two children.

Almost one half of rural caregivers (46%) were caring for children who have special needs. Most (60%) of the rural caregivers did not have their own children or any other child in their home. Twenty percent were the only adult in the home; a majority of respondents (56%) had one other adult living with them in their household. Only 25% of the caregivers indicated that the children in their care had no contact with their biological parents. Finally, 43% of respondents had been caring for their relative's child for more than 3 years.

TABLE 1 Sociodemographic Characteristics of Rural Caregivers

Caregiver characteristic	Frequency	Percent
Caregiver gender		
Male	6	10
Female	54	90
Caregiver's age (Mean age = 53; Range = 21–84)		
Younger than age 30	3	5
30–39	5	9
40–49	11	19
50–59	19	32
60–69	16	27
70+ years	5	9
Marital status		
Single	6	10
Married	26	43
Separated	6	10
Divorced	11	18
Widowed	12	20
Caregiver ethnicity		
African American	6	15
White	18	44
Latino/a American	2	5
Native American	15	37
Caregiver's yearly income		
Less than $10,000	13	22
$10,000–$20,000	25	42
$20,001–$30,000	14	23
$30,001–$40,000	3	5
$50,001–$60,000	2	3
$60,001–$70,000	0	0
More than $70,000	3	5
Caregiver's source of income		
Employment	29	54
Social Security retirement	13	24
Social Security disability	11	20
Private pension	1	2
Caregiver's educational background		
Less than high school education	8	13
General Education Diploma	8	13
High school diploma	18	30
Some college	20	33
Associate's degree	6	10
Bachelor's degree	1	2
Housing status		
Government-assisted housing	4	7
Renting	19	31
Homeowner	37	61
Living w/family or friends	4	2

Note. $N = 61$. Rounding resulted in some percent categories totaling slightly less or more than 100.

TABLE 2 Sociodemographic Characteristics of the Children in Their Care (*N* = 122)

Child characteristic	Frequency	Percent
Child's gender		
Male	47	41
Female	67	59
Ages of children:		
1–5 years of age	39	35
6–10 years of age	32	29
11–18 years of age	41	37
How many of your relative's children are you caring for		
One child	26	43
Two children	23	38
Three children	8	13
Four children	2	3
More than four children	2	3
Child's special needs status		
Yes, at least one child has one or more special needs	26	46
No, none of the children have special needs	31	54
Number of other children in the household		
None	36	60
One	11	18
Two	8	13
Three	1	2
Four	4	7
Child's contact with parent		
Regular contact	17	28
Every now and then (termed intermittent contact)	28	47
No contact	15	25
Number of years child has been in caregiver's care		
Less than a year	12	21
1–3 years	21	36
More than 3 years	25	43

Note. N = 122. Rounding resulted in some percent categories totaling slightly less or more than 100.

Study Overview and Data Collection Procedures

This university Institutional Review Board–approved study sought the impressions of kinship caregivers who lived primarily in urban, rural, and frontier portions of a large southwestern state in the United States. The results reported here are a subanalysis of a larger study (Denby, 2011, 2012) that examined the effect of a service approach called Systems of Care on kinship care. The analyses reported here are based on two research questions: (1) what are the experiences of rural kinship caregivers and (2) how do caregivers' experiences influence the well-being of the children in their care?

Caregivers interested in participating in the study completed and returned a survey instrument that was mailed to their home address. The sampling frame containing the caregivers' contact information was generated by community-based organizations and public agencies that collaborated with a university-based research team. The collaborating agencies included the lead public child welfare agency, the state Temporary Assistance to Needy Families (TANF) office, and a private nonprofit parent advocacy organization. The sampling frames were organized into groups of three types of caregivers: (1) foster care–licensed and unlicensed kinship caregivers involved with the child welfare system, (2) non-needy caretakers receiving monthly stipends from TANF, and (3) informal kinship caregivers with no involvement with any type of child and family-serving entity.

Using the Dillman total design method (Dillman, 1978; Dillman, Smyth, & Christian, 2008), the caregivers received a total of four mailings (i.e., initial survey, follow-up postcard, reminder letter, second survey) from the university over the course of a 7-week period. Also, participation was incentivized through the issuance of $25 Wal-Mart gift cards. These methods and the use of up-to-date sampling frames resulted in a 70% response rate.

Instrumentation

The Kinship in Nevada (KIN) (Denby, 2011, 2012) is a self-report, 150-item measure comprising 11 subscales: Reasons for Caring for Relative's Children, Caregiver Motivation and Sustaining Factors scale (CMSF), Caregiver Perceptions and Experiences scale (CPE), Service Needs and Community Resources, Caregiver's Perception of Children's Needs and Well-Being, Childrearing and Parenting Abilities, Caregiver Readiness and Capacity scale, Family Involvement and Social Support scale, Caregiver Strain scale, Permanency Intentions, and Caregiver, Child, and Family Characteristics. This quantitative measure resulted from a multiphase qualitative study of the experiences and perceptions of kinship caregivers. The Likert-type scaled items in the measure ranged in value from 1 (*never*) to 4 (*all of the time*). Respondents were also given a choice of *NA*. Six of the 11 subscales are reported in this analysis. On the Service Need subscale, a higher score indicates a higher level of caregiver need. On the Caregiver Readiness/Capacity and the Childrearing and Parenting Ability subscales, higher scores indicate a higher level of functioning. A high score on the Stress and Strain subscale indicates that the caregiver is experiencing a higher level of stress and strain. The Family Involvement and Social Support Scale (FISS) subscale has the same value range of 1 to 4 as the other subscales, and a higher value indicates a higher level of support. Pilot testing of the tool led to several item iterations. Reliability scores for the subscales ranged from .82 to .94. The analysis reported here resulted in recoding of variables for directionality purposes and differs from the coding described in Denby (2011).

Data Analysis

The data were analyzed using a combination of descriptive (frequencies and means) and inferential (independent sample *t* test, one-way ANOVA, correlation) statistics. Answers to research questions were sought by calculating the mean score of all the items contained in the respective subscales to generate the scale score for each respondent. Cases without valid data for at least one half of the items in each subscale were excluded from the analyses. After computing frequencies, percentages, and means, t tests were conducted for dichotomous variables and some variables were recoded into dichotomous categories to further test for significant statistical differences. For the nondichotomous variables, an ANOVA test was used to determine whether sociodemographic differences might influence the caregivers' scores on the various subscales. Finally, correlation tests, including Pearson and Spearman, were used to determine the statistical strength of the relationship between child well-being and the factors that define the caregiving experience.

FINDINGS

Indicators of Caregiver Functioning and General Experiences

Five indicators were used to determine the rural kinship caregivers' level of functioning and general experiences.

CAREGIVER READINESS AND CAPACITY

The Caregiver Readiness and Capacity subscale was designed to capture how caregivers felt about the responsibility of becoming a caregiver for their relatives' child. The mean of 3.09 is above the midpoint of the value range and indicates a high level of readiness and caregiver capacity (see Table 3). To test whether sociodemographic differences might influence caregiver readiness and capacity scores, ANOVA tests were conducted for nondichotomous variables. Additionally, t tests were conducted for

TABLE 3 Rural Caregivers' Readiness/Capacity, Ability, Stress/Strain, Family Involvement/ Support, and Needs/Resources and Child Well-Being

Scale	n	M	SD
Caregiver Readiness/Capacity	60	3.09	.49416
Childrearing/Parenting Ability	61	3.21	.42238
Caregiver Stress/Strain	60	2.03	.63744
Family Involvement/Social Support	54	2.50	.86188
Children's Needs/Well-Being	56	3.22	.33710
Service Needs	55	2.17	.58946
Community Resources (Part A)–Access, Knowledge, and Availability	55	2.50	.58994
Community Resources (Part B)–Frustration and Dissatisfaction	61	3.33	.41170

dichotomous variables. Sociodemographics did not account for differences in caregiver readiness.

CHILDREARING AND PARENTING ABILITY

The Childrearing and Parenting Ability subscale included such items as "I feel that the child (ren) and I have bonded" and "I feel that the care I am providing is making a difference in the child (ren)'s lives." The subscale resulted in a mean of 3.21, suggesting strong abilities with respect to childrearing skills and parenting. Again, to determine whether the caregivers' sociodemographics make a difference in their childrearing and parenting abilities, ANOVAs and t tests were run. There were no statistically significant differences between the various sociodemographic categories and the caregivers' childrearing and parenting abilities.

CAREGIVER STRESS AND STRAIN

On the Caregiver Stress and Strain measure, the mean scale score of the sample was 2.03, which is below the midpoint of the value range, and no respondents had a score at the highest level of the range. This indicates a relatively low level of strain. A t test was conducted to compare rural and nonrural caregivers on indicators of stress and strain and the two groups showed no statistical difference.

FAMILY INVOLVEMENT AND SOCIAL SUPPORT

The rural caregivers' family involvement and social support (FISS) scores were widely dispersed ($SD = .86$) and the mean scale score of the sample was close to the midpoint of the value range ($M = 2.50$). Such a score does suggest a high level of family involvement or social support. Additional analyses were conducted to determine if FISS scores correlate with Caregiver Readiness and Capacity and with Childrearing and Parenting Ability scores. The FISS scale strongly correlated with the readiness/capacity ($R = .540$) and childrearing/parenting abilities ($R = .558$) measure. Both positive correlations are statistically significant ($p < .01$). Further analysis was conducted to determine which of the five items in the FISS scale correlate most highly with the Capacity and Childrearing scales. The Caregiver Readiness and Capacity subscale correlated with four of five items in the FISS. It correlated most highly with Item 4 ("Neighborhood and/or community programs are a big help to us in the care of the children"; $R = .475$) and Item 3 ("My friends and/or neighbors are a big support in the care of the children"; $R = .404$). The Childrearing and Parenting Ability scale correlated with all five items of the FISS. It correlated most highly with Item 4 ("Neighborhood and/or community programs are a big help to us in the care of the children"; $R = .522$) and Item 5 ("Networking with other relative caregivers is a big support to me"; $R = .512$).

SERVICE NEEDS AND COMMUNITY RESOURCES

Two scales were used to measure the caregivers' service needs and their access to community resources. Combined, the two scales contain 33 items. High scores on the Service Needs subscale indicate that the caregivers have identified a high level of need and that they feel they could benefit from a range of service options that are associated with the caregiving experience. As an extension of the Service Needs subscale, the Community Resources scale measures the extent to which caregivers report that their needs are being addressed through the provision of community services. The Community Resources subscale has two parts: (1) caregivers' report of access, availability, and knowledge of community resources and (2) caregivers' report of frustration experienced while trying to acquire services and supports on behalf of the children in their care.

The mean on the Service Needs subscale was 2.17, which suggests that rural caregivers are mostly having their needs met. With respect to the second scale, the Community Resources measure, the range is from 1 to 4, where a higher score in the access, availability, and knowledge portion of the scale signifies that the caregiver is not experiencing great difficulty knowing where and how to get services; however, a higher score in the second part of the measure indicates a high level of frustration during the service delivery process. The Community Resources (Part A) scale resulted in a mean of 2.50, which may show that the rural caregivers have some knowledge of services and how to access them; however, Part B's mean was 3.33, which indicates a high level of frustration or dissatisfaction during the service delivery process. We conducted t tests to compare rural to nonrural caregivers on service needs and their experiences with community resources. Although there was no difference between rural and nonrural caregivers on how highly they rated their need for services, there was a statistically significant ($p < .05$) difference in Part A of the Community Resources subscale. Rural caregivers had a 7% lower score on their self-rating of access, availability, and knowledge of community resources. In other words, although the rural kinship caregivers expressed some degree of knowledge about the availability of resources and how to access them, nonrural kinship caregivers find that they are more knowledgeable and more likely to access available services. The two groups did not differ in their reports of frustration and dissatisfaction once engaged in or receiving services; both groups reported high levels of frustration.

Child Well-Being

The Children's Needs and Well-being subscale contained questions that positioned the caregiver to register his or her perceptions about the emotional health and mental health conditions of the child in his or her care. Sample items include, "The children say they feel strange or embarrassed around other children because they live with us and not their parents" and "I feel that the children need counseling." The mean scale score of the sample was 3.22 out of 4.0, which is well above the midpoint of the value range, and no respondents had a mean score at either of the two lowest values of the range. This suggests a high level of perceived child well-being. We used t tests and correlations to explore whether sociodemographic differences might influence scores on the Children's Needs and Well-being scale. None of the sociodemographic variables demonstrated any statistically significant differences between groups. Differences in income, age, education, ethnicity, gender, marital status, number of adults in the household, and housing type did not correspond to differences on the Well-Being scale. Nor were there correlations between the scale score and age or income. Additionally, an analysis was conducted to determine if other relevant scales correlated with the Children's Needs and Well-Being subscale. Four of the five scales did have statistically significant correlations with the well-being scale, with the Family Involvement and Social Support subscale being the exception. The scale that correlates most highly is the caregiver Stress and Strain measure ($R = -.350$, $p < .01$). This negative correlation means a higher Stress and Strain score is predictive of a lower Children's Needs and Well-Being score. Other scales that correlated negatively were Service Needs ($R = -.337$, $p < .05$) and Community Resources (Part B) ($R = -.296$, $p < .05$), which means that respondents who expressed a higher service need and frustration and dissatisfaction with services had lower perceived child well-being. Caregiver Readiness and Capacity ($R = .340$, $p = .05$) and Childrearing and Parenting Ability ($R = .302$, $p = .05$) are predictive of higher perceived child well-being.

DISCUSSION

The rural caregivers in this sample were like most other caregivers. They were largely low-income women who had earned a high school diploma or GED. Findings associated with limited financial resources and less education are corroborated by others who have studied this population (see Bullock, 2007; King et al., 2009; Radel, Bramlett, & Waters, 2010; Sakai, Lin, & Flores, 2011). However, these rural caregivers did differ slightly from the typical caregiver profile in that many of them described their ethnic background as Native American. Also, slightly different from the traditional profile, these rural caregivers tended to be homeowners, and although there was a full range of age groups, the average age was only 53, indicating a younger cohort than observed in many studies of kinship caregivers. The caregivers reported limited financial resources but high readiness and capacity to parent. Likewise, the caregivers did not exhibit high levels of stress and strain; their scores were somewhat moderate.

Such findings may indicate that these rural caregivers possess remarkable strengths and abilities despite the caregiving challenges that they faced. Indeed, other research has also noted the parenting strengths of rural kinship caregivers. For example, in research by Sheridan, Haight, and Cleeland (2011) it was found that for rural children exposed to methamphetamine-addicted parents, grandparent caregivers were likely to buffer feelings of aggression and decrease problematic behavior by acting as positive role models.

Part of what may contribute to the rural caregivers' strengths and capacities is family involvement and social support. Many of the caregivers indicated high levels of family involvement and social support and those who did possess this resource were also the ones who exhibited the highest scores on caregiver readiness/capacity and parenting abilities. What seems to help most is the presence of community programs, outlets, and opportunities to network with other caregivers and friends and neighbors who are available to help out with the children. Other researchers have also noted the profoundly positive effect that social supports have on kinship caregivers (Sands & Goldberg-Glen, 2000; Smith, Savage-Stevens, & Fabian, 2002).

In terms of needs and challenges, we found that the caregivers identified a minimum level of needs. However, as it relates to knowledge of services and the ability to access the same, nonrural caregivers had an advantage. Additionally, the rural caregivers reported extremely high levels of frustration and dissatisfaction with the service delivery process and their receipt of services. Other research has also found that knowledge of and access to services is a significant problem for caregivers (King at al., 2009; Kropf & Kolomer, 2004; Letiecq et al., 2008; Myers et al., 2002). The rural caregivers' experiences with services were significant because there was a direct correlation between the children's well-being and the caregivers' perception of whether their service needs were being met. Those caregivers with the highest service needs and highest levels of frustration when attempting to acquire services were the caregivers whose children's well-being scores were the lowest. In addition to service needs, the other conditions that influenced how the children being cared for by rural caregivers fare included stress and strain and the caregivers' perceptions of their readiness and their parenting abilities. Higher caregiver stress and strain scores predicted low child well-being scores. Moreover, children whose caregivers scored lowest in the rating of readiness/capacity and childrearing abilities/parenting had the lowest well-being markers. These findings contribute to what is known about the effect of unmet service needs on rural kinship caregivers. These data may suggest that unmet service needs negatively affect children's well-being, and Letiecq et al. (2008) found that the effect is also experienced by the caregiver. Specifically, Letiecq et al. discovered that rural grandparent caregivers' mental health is likely to be compromised due to "a lack of jobs, food insecurity, and a lack of child care" (p. 338).

The findings here, combined with what we already know about rural caregiving, rural living, and kinship care in general, justify a unique education and practice approach aimed at increasing practitioners' effectiveness with rural families. To recap, previous research informs us that kinship children in rural areas may experience difficulties transitioning because of unfamiliarity with the area (Kropf & Kolomer, 2004) or issues associated with rural life (Heflinger & Hoffman, 2009). Additionally, we know that children in kinship care are less likely to receive treatment for health concerns (Schneiderman & Villagrana, 2010) and are generally found to be in poorer health (Radel et al., 2010) than children in nonrelative foster care. Also, children growing up in rural kinship care placements may be at an increased risk because of higher rates of child poverty, which is associated with a greater likelihood of poor health and child maltreatment (Belanger & Stone, 2008). Finally, Starr et al. (2002) explained, "many conditions identified as risk factors for the development of child and adolescent mental health problems, such as poverty, family disruptions, including single parent households, and poor employment opportunities are prevalent in rural communities" (p. 293).

Limitations

The limitations of this study are the small sample size, the use of self-reports, and the cross-sectional nature of the design. For example, in several of the tests that sought to measure group differences, we were unable to detect statistically significant results. This is likely due to the relatively small sample size. Also, the limitations associated with the use of self-report, including social desirability of responses and positive self-perceptions (Cook & Campbell, 1979), and accuracy of recall (Schacter, 1999) are applicable in this study. This was a cross-sectional study that discovered several significant correlations between child well-being and conditions experienced by caregivers. However, readers are reminded that correlational findings should not be interpreted as causal findings.

Implications

Very limited education about interventions with kinship caregiver families is provided in social work and even less information is provided about practice approaches with rural families. Therefore, it is important to equip future practitioners with information that will help them address the needs of kinship caregivers in order for the caregivers to better understand how to assist the children living in their care.

EDUCATION AND PRACTICE STRATEGIES

Attribution theory provides a useful lens through which to interpret the findings of this study and to understand plausible practice directions. When making attributions for why children's well-being status may not be optimal, kinship caregivers face a set of circumstances unique to their position. Indeed, kinship caregivers in rural regions are also likely to experience concerns different from those of other caregivers. For example, kinship caregivers may be more inclined to care for their relatives' children in voluntary or informal arrangements that do not allow for the same rights and services (e.g., government assistance and the right to consent on behalf of the children) as foster parents in formal foster care arrangements (Child Welfare Information Gateway, 2010). The literature reports that rural kinship caregivers express a need for legal support (Myers et al., 2002), as many rural grandparents express fear of losing custody of their grandchildren (King et al., 2009; Myers et al., 2002); however, a mistrust of government is common among rural caregivers (Bullock, 2007), which may impede the formalizing process.

What this means is that practitioners may need to expand their understanding of attribution theory's notion of self-serving bias as it relates to rural kinship caregivers. Such an understanding begins during the practitioner's education and training. Coursework that prepares students to possess sound engagement and assessment skills is critical. It is helpful for practitioners to understand that rural kinship caregivers may require a carefully planned engagement period during which a high level of trust is established. The children in their care may be experiencing tremendous unmet needs, and the caregivers could lack the capacity to address those needs, but the caregivers may be guarded with such disclosures.

POLICIES AND PROGRAMMING STRATEGIES

Social workers and other mental health professionals can focus on methods of improving the outcomes experienced by children in rural kinship caregiver arrangements by pursuing policy advocacy that addresses service provision differentials. Targeted funding to community-based organizations that provide outreach to rural families is one type of policy and legislative goal that could be pursued by advocates. Additionally, increased attention to the needs of rural kinship caregivers can occur by the issuance of federal demonstration projects that prioritize the development of initiatives to support the uncommon needs of this population. Finally, social workers can assist rural kinship caregiver families by helping to forge community collaboratives and provider networks to establish social support networks to augment formal service delivery structures.

SUMMARY AND CONCLUSION

The challenges associated with caring for relatives' children and rearing them in rural environments may pose service needs that many social service professionals are not trained to address. This exploratory study determined that children living in rural kinship care arrangements are perceived to have low levels of well-being when their caregivers are experiencing unmet service needs, high levels of stress and strain, low childrearing and parenting abilities, and low levels of capacity and readiness. Future research using larger sample sizes can expand our level of understanding about the specific level of capacity, readiness, and childrearing abilities that rural kinship caregivers need in order for them to perceive that the children in their care are enjoying high levels of well-being. Also, studies that are able to manipulate conditions and employ comparison samples could possibly shed light on the causal relationship between indicators of child well-being and provision of services. Understanding the uniqueness of rural kinship caregivers helps us to assess the complexity of their situations so that we are able to assist them in supporting the needs of the children in their care.

ACKNOWLEDGMENTS

We wish to thank all of the individuals who devoted time to the data collection and analysis efforts that supported the development of this article, including: Chris Kordus, Constance Brooks, Renee Brown, Nancy Downey, and Nickolas Liebman.

REFERENCES

Belanger, K., & Stone, W. (2008). The social service divide: Service availability and accessibility in rural versus urban counties and impact on child welfare outcomes. *Child Welfare, 87*(4), 101–124.

Bullock, K. (2007). Grandfathers raising grandchildren: An exploration of African American kinship networks. *Journal of Health & Social Policy, 22*(3/4), 181–197. doi:10.1300/J045v22n03_12

Campbell, W. K., & Sedikides, C. (1999). Self-threat magnifies the self-serving bias: A meta-analytic integration. *Review of General Psychology, 3*(1), 23–43.

Child Welfare Information Gateway, Administration on Children, Youth and Families, Children's Bureau. (2010). *Kinship caregivers and the child welfare system.* Retrieved from http://www.childwelfare.gov/pubs/f_kinshi/

Conklin, C. (1980). Rural community care-givers. *Social Work, 25*(6), 495–496.

Cook, T. D., & Campbell, D. T. (1979). *Quasi-experimentation: Design and analysis issues.* Boston, MA: Houghton Mifflin.

Denby, R. W. (2011). Predicting permanency intentions among kinship caregivers. *Child and Adolescent Social Work Journal, 28*(2), 113–131.

Denby, R. W. (2012). Parental incarceration and kinship care: Caregiver experiences, child well-being and permanency intentions. *Journal of Social Work and Public Health, 27*(1/2), 104–128.

Dillman, D. A. (1978). *Mail and telephone surveys: The total design method.* New York, NY: Wiley.

Dillman, D. A., Smyth, J. D., & Christian, L. M. (2008). *Internet, mail and mixed-mode surveys: The tailored design method* (3rd ed.). New York, NY: Wiley.

Gilbert, D. T. (1998). Speeding with Ned: A personal view of the correspondence bias. In J. M. Darley & J. Cooper (Ed.), *Attribution and social interaction: The legacy of Edward E. Jones* (pp. 5–36). Washington, DC: American Psychological Association.

Gilovich, T. (1987). Secondhand information and social judgment. *Journal of Experimental Social Psychology, 23,* 59–74.

Heflinger, C. A., & Hoffman, C. (2009). Double whammy? Rural youth with serious emotional disturbance and the transition to adulthood. *Journal of Rural Health, 25*(4), 399–406.

Heider, F. (1958). *The psychology of interpersonal relations.* New York, NY: Wiley.

Ichheiser, G. (1943). Misinterpretations of personality in everyday life and the psychologist's frame of reference. *Character and Personality, 12,* 145–160.

King, S., Kropf, N. P., Perkins, M., Sessley, L., Burt, C., & Lepore, M. (2009). Kinship care in rural Georgia communities: Responding to needs and challenges of grandparent caregivers. *Journal of Intergenerational Relationships, 7*(2/3), 225–242. doi:10.1080/15350770902852369

Kropf, N. P., & Kolomer, S. (2004). Grandparents raising grandchildren: A diverse population. *Journal of Human Behavior in the Social Environment, 9*(4), 65–83. doi:10.1300/J137v09n04_04

Larson, N. C., & Dearmont, M. (2002). Strengths of farming communities in fostering resilience in children. *Child Welfare, 81*(5), 821–835.

Lauver, L. S. (2010). The lived experience of foster parents of children with special needs living in rural areas. *Journal of Pediatric Nursing, 25*(4), 289–298.

Letiecq, B. L., Bailey, S. J., & Kurtz, M. A. (2008). Depression among rural Native American and European American grandparents rearing their grandchildren. *Journal of Family Issues, 29*(3), 334–356.

McGuinness, T. M. (2009). Almost invisible: Rural youth in foster care. *Journal of Child and Adolescent Psychiatric Nursing, 22*(2), 55–56. doi:10.1111/j.1744-6171.2009.00172.x

Miller, D. T., & Ross, R. (1975). Self-serving biases in the attribution of causality: Fact or fiction? *Psychological Bulletin, 82*(2), 213–225.

Myers, L. L., Kropf, N. P., & Robinson, M. (2002). Grandparents raising grandchildren: Case management in a rural setting. *Journal of Human Behavior in the Social Environment, 5*(1), 53–71.

Radel, L. F., Bramlett, M. D., & Waters, A. (2010). Legal and informal adoption by relatives in the U.S.: Comparative characteristics and well-being from a nationally representative sample. *Adoption Quarterly, 13*(3/4), 268–291.

Sakai, C., Lin, H., & Flores, G. (2011). Health outcomes and family services in kinship care: Analysis of a national sample of children in the child welfare system. *Archives of Pediatrics & Adolescent Medicine, 165*(2), 159–165.

Salkind, N. J. (2005). Attribution theory. In *Encyclopedia of human development.* Thousand Oaks: Sage. doi:10.4135/9781412952484

Sands, R. G., & Goldberg-Glen, R. S. (2000). Factors associated with stress among grandparents raising their grandchildren. *Family Relations, 49*(1), 97–105.

Schacter, D. L. (1999). The seven sins of memory: Insights from psychology and cognitive neuroscience. *American Psychology, 54*, 182–203.

Schneiderman, J. U., & Villagrana, M. (2010). Meeting children's mental and physical health needs in child welfare: The importance of caregivers. *Social Work in Health Care, 49*(2), 91–108.

Shepperd, J., Malone, W., & Sweeny, K. (2008). Exploring causes of the self-serving bias. *Social and Personality Psychology Compass, 2*(2), 895–908.

Sheridan, K., Haight, W. L., & Cleeland, L. (2011). The role of grandparents in preventing aggressive and other externalizing behavior problems in children from rural, methamphetamine-involved families. *Children and Youth Services Review, 33*(9), 1583–1591. doi:10.1016/j.childyouth.2011.03.023

Smith, G. C., Savage-Stevens, S. E., & Fabian, E. S. (2002). How caregiving grandparents view support groups for grandchildren in their care. *Family Relations, 51*(3), 274–281.

Starr, S., Campbell, L. R., & Herrick, C. A. (2002). Factors affecting use of the mental health system by rural children. *Issues in Mental Health Nursing, 23*(29), 291–304.

U.S. Census Bureau, American Community Survey. (2006–2010). *Percent of grandparents responsible for their grandchildren* (GCT 1001). Retrieved from American Fact Finder: http://factfinder2.census.gov/faces/tableservices/jsf/pages/product view.xhtml?pid=ACS_10_5YR_GCT1001.US26&prodType=table

U.S. Census Bureau, Geography Division. (2012). *2010 Census urban and rural classification and urban area criteria.* Retrieved from http://www.census.gov/geo/www/ua/2010urbanruralclass.html

U.S. Department of Health and Human Services, Health Resources and Services Administration. (2011). *The health and well-being of children in rural areas: A portrait of the nation 2007.* Rockville, MD: U.S. Department of Health and Human Services.

Weiner, B. (1986). *An attributional theory of motivation and emotion.* New York, NY: Springer-Verlag.

Preventing Adolescent Risk Behavior in the Rural Context: An Integrative Analysis of Adolescent, Parent, and Provider Perspectives

CARRIE W. RISHEL

School of Social Work, West Virginia University, Morgantown, West Virginia

LESLEY COTTRELL

Department of Pediatrics, West Virginia University, Morgantown, West Virginia

TRICIA KINGERY

West Virginia Child Care Association, Charleston, West Virginia

Adolescent risk behavior remains prevalent and contributes to numerous social problems and growing health care costs. Contrary to popular perception, adolescents in rural areas engage in risky behaviors at least as much as youth from urban or suburban settings. Little research, however, focuses on risk behavior prevention in the rural context. This study integrates adolescent, parent, and provider perspectives related to adolescent risk behavior engagement and prevention to suggest promising prevention strategies for rural families and communities.

Contrary to popular stereotypes of idyllic rural environments, research suggests that adolescents in rural settings may be more likely to engage in risky behaviors than their urban and suburban counterparts (Atav & Spencer, 2002; Puskar, Tusaie-Mumford, Sereika, & Lamb, 1999). As defined by the Centers for Disease Control and Prevention (CDC), adolescent risk behaviors include specific behaviors that contribute to major health problems (Kolbe, Kann, & Collins, 1993). About 80% of the West Virginia population resides in rural communities (Economic Research Service [ERS], 2012). Based on data from the Youth Risk Behavior Survey, higher percentages of adolescents in West

Virginia report engaging in risk behaviors such as cigarette smoking (59% WV vs. 50% USA), binge drinking (30% WV vs. 26% USA), marijuana use (41% WV vs. 38% USA), cocaine use (11% WV vs. 7% USA), sexual intercourse (54% WV vs. 48% USA), and sexual intercourse with four or more partners (17% WV vs. 15% USA) than the national average (CDC, 2009). Although rural adolescents often experience high levels of risk factors such as social isolation, early drug and alcohol use, and early sexual initiation, the majority of adolescent risk behavior research has focused on urban youth with less attention to rural adolescents (Dunn et al., 2008). With available treatment programs generally few and far between in rural areas, prevention interventions appropriate to the rural context are critically needed to decrease risk behavior engagement among rural adolescents.

This study is informed by the risk and protective factor model, which is recognized as the best available framework for the prevention of adolescent health and behavioral problems (Hawkins, Catalano, & Arthur, 2002). *Risk factors* are defined as circumstances in an adolescent's life that increase the likelihood of negative outcomes (Durlak, 1998; Smith & Carlson, 1997), whereas *protective factors* refer to circumstances that decrease the likelihood of negative outcomes for that adolescent (Durlak, 1998). Risk and protective factors are typically categorized into three groups: individual factors, family factors, and environmental factors (Garmezy, 1985). This study examines factors at the family and environmental levels that have been linked to adolescent risk behavior. The terms *adolescent risk behavior* and *adolescent risk involvement* are used interchangeably in this study, with *adolescent risk involvement* referring to adolescent engagement in risk behaviors.

Family-level factors considered in this study include parent–adolescent communication, parental monitoring, and parental substance abuse. Parent–adolescent communication has been clearly linked to adolescent risk behavior (Guilamo-Ramos, Jaccard, Dittus, & Bouris, 2006), with multiple studies demonstrating that warm, supportive, and open parent–adolescent communication protects against youth risk behavior (Hawkins, Catalano, & Miller, 1992; Kafka & London, 1991). More specifically, direct communication between adolescents and their parents regarding specific risk behaviors and consequences is associated with less adolescent risk involvement (Diaz et al., 2006; Miller, Burgoon, Grandpre, & Alvaro, 2006). Parental monitoring is another family-level factor shown to protect against multiple areas of adolescent risk (Stanton et al., 2000). Specifically, increased parental monitoring has been associated with significantly less engagement in adolescent risk behavior (Howard, Qiu, & Boekeloo, 2003; Rai et al., 2003) and has been demonstrated to predict lower adolescent risk involvement in the future (King & Chassin, 2004; Li, Feigelman, & Stanton, 2000; Rai et al., 2003; Wu et al., 2003). Finally, parental substance abuse has also been linked to negative health outcomes for adolescents. More specifically, children of substance abusing parents are at increased risk of abusing substances themselves

(Francis, 2011) and have higher rates of behavioral problems and substance use than children of parents with no history of substance abuse (Merikangas, Dierker, & Szatmari, 1998).

Environmental-level factors considered in this study include adolescent relationships with nonparental adults, academic achievement, and the prevalence of norms and values that support risky behavior. Supportive relationships with nonparental adults have been clearly associated with positive developmental outcomes for adolescents (Garmezy, 1985; Rishel, Sales, & Koeske, 2005; Werner, 1992, 1995). More specifically, Greenberger, Chen, and Beam (1998) found that adolescents who report a strong relationship with a "very important" nonparental adult are less likely to engage in risky behaviors. Adolescents who develop strong, positive relationships with nonparental adults are also less likely to exhibit behavior problems than other adolescents (Rishel et al., 2005). Academic achievement, a school-related environmental factor, is also significantly associated with adolescent risk behavior. For example, Sullivan, Childs, and O'Connell (2010) found that lower school grades were significantly associated with higher risk behavior engagement across a range of risky behaviors including substance use and sexual risk behaviors. Finally, community norms are another environmental-level variable shown to be associated with youth risk behavior. Recent research demonstrates that parent, peer, and community norms are related to adolescent substance use (Song, Smiler, Wagner, & Wolfson, 2012), and perceived peer norms around safer sexual practices are related to sexual risk taking behavior among adolescents (Kapaia et al., 2012).

This study uses data from a sample of adolescents and parents in a rural setting to examine family and community correlates of adolescent risk behavior. These findings are then compared to rural youth service provider perspectives regarding the development and prevention of adolescent risk behavior in a rural context. The purpose of this study is to address three research questions: (1) What family and community factors specific to the rural context are shown to be associated with adolescent risk behavior? (2) Do adolescents, parents, and providers agree on the rural factors associated with adolescent risk behavior? and (3) What promising prevention strategies emerge for rural settings that should be pursued in future efforts?

METHOD

Data from two separate studies were used in this investigation. The first study was initially conducted in 2005 and included data collection from parents and adolescents from across the state of West Virginia. Further details on the methodology of this study can be found in previous publications (Rishel et al., 2007; Rishel, Cottrell, Stanton, Cottrell, & Branstetter, 2010). Additional analyses of data collected in this study were conducted for the current investigation. The second study was conducted in 2010 and included data collection from youth service providers across the state. The analysis of this data has not been reported elsewhere.

Study 1

The first study included 518 parent–adolescent dyads recruited from 32 rural middle and high schools across the state of West Virginia to participate in a longitudinal study exploring parental monitoring and related issues. Baseline questionnaire responses from parents and adolescents addressing family and community factors as related to adolescent risk involvement were used for this study. Adolescent and parent forms were linked for analyses through a unique identifier created for each family. All procedures were approved by the Institutional Review Board at West Virginia University. The average age of the adolescent sample was 15 years (range 12–17 years, $SD = 1.3$), and that of participating parents was 41 years ($SD = 6.78$). The majority of adolescents (70%, $n = 363$) and parents (91%, $n = 473$) were female, and almost all families identified themselves as White (96%, $n = 496$), reflecting the racial composition of the state. More than one third of participating adolescents (37%, $n = 190$) reported substance use in the past four months including alcohol (31%), tobacco (19%), marijuana (10%), and other drugs (7%). Likewise, more than one third of participating adolescents (34%, $n = 174$) reported being sexually active within the past 4 months.

Study 2

The second study included a survey of 440 adolescent service providers from across West Virginia focused on identifying factors that contribute to adolescent risk behavior and possible prevention strategies. The anonymous survey was developed and distributed through the West Virginia Child Care Association, an organization that represents companies that operate behavioral health and child welfare programs statewide. The West Virginia Child Care Association implemented the provider survey as the first step in a multi-year project aimed at developing an at-risk prevention outreach and training series for youth-serving professionals throughout the state. Survey questions addressed provider perceptions regarding contributing factors to adolescent risk behavior, current prevention and training efforts within provider organizations, and how specific stakeholder groups could contribute to better prevention of youth risk behavior. The survey was distributed online through Survey Monkey and completed by a variety of youth service providers including social service workers, probation officers, juvenile court officers, child welfare caseworkers, teachers, administrators, and school counselors. The majority of survey questions instructed respondents to "choose up to three" out of multiple choices, resulting in mostly descriptive analyses of responses. All procedures were approved by the Institutional Review Board at West Virginia University.

Data Analysis

Using data from Study 1, bivariate correlations and independent sample t tests were used to examine relationships between adolescent risk behavior and four factors shown to be related to adolescent risk behavior: parent–adolescent communication, parental monitoring, adolescents' relationships with nonparental adults, and school grades. The correlations of adolescent risk behavior with parent–adolescent communication, parental monitoring, and adolescent relationships with nonparental adults have been previously published in separate reports that are cited as appropriate. These findings, along with a current analysis of the association of school grades and adolescent risk behavior, are summarized under the report of results for Research Question 1.

To address Research Question 2, descriptive analyses were conducted using data collected in Study 2 to rank provider responses on survey questions addressing the four factors examined in this study. To determine agreement on these factors, the provider responses are then compared to the adolescent and parent report.

To address Research Question 3, provider responses regarding specific prevention strategies for the rural context were examined. Survey items examined included provider perspectives regarding current prevention and training efforts within their organizations, the most frequently identified ways in which providers thought specific stakeholders should be involved in prevention efforts, and provider responses regarding specific agency strategies to strengthen community-wide prevention efforts.

RESULTS

Research Question 1: Family and Community Correlates of Rural Risk

Of the four factors examined in this study, parent–adolescent communication and school grades appear to be the factors most strongly associated with adolescent risk behavior in this rural sample. Based on research conducted in 2010 by Rishel et al., adolescents who reported more positive communication with parents also reported significantly less engagement in risk behavior ($r = -.36$, $p < .05$). More specifically, adolescents who reported more comfort in conversing about risk behaviors report significantly less engagement in risk behavior ($r = -.29$, $p < .05$). It is interesting to note that parent-reported comfort in conversing about risk behaviors was not significantly related to adolescent report of risk behavior engagement (Ice &

Cottrell, 2010). Parent report also indicated that adolescents who received higher grades in school (mostly As and Bs) were less likely than adolescents who received lower grades to engage in risky behaviors ($t = -4.45$; $p < .05$).

Somewhat surprisingly, subscales measuring "direct" and "indirect" parental monitoring were not significantly associated with adolescent risk behavior in this sample of rural adolescents. "Direct" monitoring strategies include parental behavior such as talking directly to adolescents about their whereabouts and activities, whereas "indirect" strategies include parental behaviors such as meeting their adolescent's friends and talking to other parents (Cottrell et al., 2007). Adolescents who reported higher levels of parental "school monitoring," also reported significantly less engagement in risk behaviors ($r = -.10$; $p < .05$). The subscale measuring school monitoring includes parental behaviors such as checking on homework, talking to teachers, and talking to their adolescent about schoolwork. Interestingly, parental report of school monitoring was not significantly related to adolescent report of risk behavior engagement (Cottrell et al., 2007).

As reported in Rishel et al. (2010), adolescents who reported stronger relationships with nonparental adults also reported less engagement in risk behavior ($r = -.15$, $p < .05$). In a previous study with this sample, authors also found that strong relationships with nonparental adults buffered the relationship of poor parent–adolescent communication and adolescent risk behavior, providing further support of the positive impact of nonparental adults in association with youth engagement in risky behaviors (Rishel et al., 2010). It is interesting to note that adolescents report significantly stronger relationships with related adults but weaker relationships with nonrelated adults than their parents perceive. The category of teacher, however, may be an exception as adolescents report especially strong relationships with their favorite teachers (Rishel et al., 2007).

Research Question 2: Comparison of Family and Provider Perspectives

To determine if provider perspectives regarding factors related to adolescent engagement in risk behavior parallel adolescent and parent report, data from the 440 statewide service providers were examined.

FAMILY FACTOR COMPARISON

When asked to choose the top three family characteristics perceived to contribute to youth risk behavior, providers most frequently cited "lack of parental monitoring" as a key contributing factor (84%, $n = 368$). The second most frequently chosen factor in the area of family characteristics was "parental substance abuse" (67%, $n = 295$), with "poor parent–child communication" the third most frequently chosen factor (38%, $n = 166$). When comparing these responses to adolescent and parent data, there is a clear difference in perspectives. Providers overwhelmingly chose lack of parental monitoring as a key contributing family characteristic to adolescent risk behavior. Parent and adolescent report, however, suggests that parent–adolescent communication is a stronger influence than parental monitoring on adolescent risk behavior, a factor that providers list as a distant third. Providers also frequently identify parental substance abuse as a key contributing family characteristic to youth risk behavior. Because the parent–adolescent survey used in this study did not inquire about parental substance abuse, the authors were unable to draw any conclusions regarding provider and family concordance on this factor.

ENVIRONMENTAL FACTOR COMPARISON

When asked to identify key school or community characteristics perceived to lead to adolescent risk behavior, providers most frequently chose the option of "poor student–teacher relationships" (47%, $n = 207$). The other two most commonly chosen factors were "poor academic achievement" (42%, $n = 183$) and "the prevalence of norms or values that support risky behaviors" (41%, $n = 178$). As noted above, previous work with the parent–adolescent sample demonstrates that youth report particularly strong relationships with "favorite teachers," supporting provider perception of the importance of student–teacher relationships. Provider perception of the link between poor academic achievement and risk behavior engagement is also supported by data from the parent–adolescent sample, which indicates that adolescents with lower grades were more likely to report engaging in risky behaviors. The parent–adolescent survey used in this study did not capture "the prevalence of norms or values that support risky behaviors," limiting the authors' ability to assess family and provider concordance on this factor.

Research Question 3: Identifying Promising Prevention Strategies for the Rural Context

In response to questions regarding current prevention and training efforts within provider organizations, one-half of respondents (50%, $n = 220$) indicated that they and their organization spend more time addressing risk behavior after it manifests, as compared to one-third (31%, $n = 136$) who indicated about equal amount of time spent on prevention and addressing the behavior after it manifests, and a minority (19%, $n = 83$) who indicated more time was spent on prevention. The majority of respondents (57%, $n = 250$) stated that they had received no professional training in prevention of youth risk behavior. Despite the lack of training and attention given to prevention within providers' current organizations, almost all providers (96%, $n = 422$) reported their belief that youth risk behavior could be prevented with intervention prior to behavior manifestation. This almost unanimous response suggests that providers within a rural context would be receptive to participating in future prevention efforts.

The top suggestions supported by providers for key stakeholder groups to assist in the prevention of youth risk behavior included parents should "actively communicate with their children" (74%, $n = 324$); schools should train school staff in the prevention of risk behavior (60%, $n = 263$); community and business leaders should establish school—community partnerships (64%, $n = 282$); social service agencies should implement, evaluate, and revise a comprehensive prevention plan (66%, $n = 292$); courts should better support youth who experience high family conflict such as domestic violence and divorce (45%, $n = 197$); and elected officials and government agencies should build collaboration among federal, state, and local agencies to pool resources and maximize use of effective approaches to the prevention of youth risk behavior (68%, $n = 297$).

When asked how agencies could better work together to prevent youth risk behavior, the three most frequently chosen responses pointed to the need for better coordination among agencies: coordinate prevention programs (69%, $n = 303$), share information (63%, $n = 277$), and coordinate training programs (50%, $n = 220$). When asked about involvement of specific stakeholder groups, providers indicated that parents (85%, $n = 375$) and teachers (71%, $n = 310$) are the most important people to train to respond to youth risk behavior, supporting the importance of relationships with parents and teachers as demonstrated in the adolescent and parent report data. Although parents and teachers are identified by providers as the most important people to train, the majority of providers (64%, $n = 280$) named community and business leaders as those they would most like to see more involved in prevention (as compared to educators, law enforcement, juvenile justice, federal, state, and social service agencies), suggesting the need for broad community involvement in developing and implementing prevention efforts.

DISCUSSION

The main goal of this study was to integrate data from adolescents, parents, and providers to identify promising prevention strategies of adolescent risk behavior for rural families and communities. The two studies used in this investigation utilized statewide samples of different categories of informants who responded to survey questions related to adolescent risk behavior. Although not perfectly comparable, the similar focus of these two studies creates an opportunity to integrate multiple viewpoints of the same issue. The synthesis of these multiple perspectives provides stronger information to guide rural community prevention efforts than would be available by solely examining these studies separately. Recommendations for promising prevention strategies that should be considered by rural communities are provided below.

Recommendations

IMPROVE PARENT–ADOLESCENT COMMUNICATION

Analyses of parent and adolescent report indicate that parent–child communication is strongly associated with youth risk behavior engagement. This is supported by provider perception of family factors related to adolescent risk behavior. Rural communities may want to consider programs aimed at strengthening communication between adolescents and parents. Programs should emphasize increasing adolescent perceived comfort in conversing about risk behaviors with their parents, as this is shown to be significantly related to risk behavior engagement. One possibility for rural communities is The Strengthening Families Program (SFP), a family-based comprehensive prevention program aimed at strengthening parenting skills, increasing positive family communication and bonding, and decreasing youth problem behaviors (Kumpfer, Alvarado, Tait, & Turner, 2002). The SFP has been shown to be effective in 15 replication studies with cultural adaptions for families of various cultural groups (Kumpfer, Alvarado, Smith, & Bellamny, 2002), has positive 5-year follow-up results, and demonstrates economic viability, with $9.60 saved for every $1 spent on the families (Kumpfer, Alvarado, & Whiteside, 2003; Spoth, Guyll, & Day, 2002). Most importantly for rural communities, the SFP has been specifically adapted for and tested with rural families (Kumpfer, Alvarado, Tait, et al., 2002).

STRENGTHEN TEACHER–STUDENT RELATIONSHIPS

Report from adolescents, their parents, and providers all indicate that youth relationships with teachers are especially important. Rural communities and schools may want to consider strategies to strengthen teacher–student relationships. One way to do this may be to implement a teacher–student mentoring program, so that each student has a "formalized" connection with at least one teacher that goes beyond the standard classroom relationship. Another strategy is to implement school-wide positive behavior supports (SWPBS), which is supported by a growing body of evidence demonstrating positive effects of SWPBS in reducing student problem behaviors (Eber, Hyde, & Suter, 2011). Recent work examining positive behavior support (PBS) strategies indicates that the clear classroom management practices utilized in PBS and SWPBS create a positive learning environment that strengthens student–teacher relationships (Sugai & Horner, 2008).

INCREASE PARENT AND COMMUNITY INVOLVEMENT IN SCHOOL

Adolescent report indicates that higher parental involvement in school is related to significantly less youth risk behavior engagement. Provider responses not only highlight the importance of parents and teachers in the prevention of adolescent risk behavior, but also point to community and business leaders as needing to play a larger role in prevention efforts. Drawing from provider responses to qualitative items regarding rural area service needs, rural communities may want to consider ways in which local schools can serve as a "hub" for prevention and early intervention services related to youth risk behavior. Multiple provider respondents offered similar suggestions, stating that the schools are "the hub of small communities within our counties" and that locating community services within the schools would alleviate transportation problems and other barriers to rural service access. This suggestion is supported by other research examining community context as related to youth risk behavior. Authors of a recent study using a large rural sample of 28 communities report that school context was the most consistently associated construct with adolescent problem behaviors. Conclusions drawn from this study highlight the importance of district leadership that emphasizes school-family relationships and parent engagement as a way to reinforce positive messages for adolescents (Chilenski & Greenberg, 2009). Intentionally utilizing rural schools as a "hub" for youth and family services may be one way to strengthen family engagement with schools, as well as promote involvement of community leaders and services in programs located within the school environment.

PROVIDE PREVENTION TRAINING

As more than one-half of provider respondents in this rural state had received no formal training on prevention, collaborative community prevention plans should include methods for training various stakeholder groups in prevention of youth risk behavior. The work of the West Virginia Child Care Association (WVCCA) can serve as an example of how this might be done in rural states and communities. The WVCCA is using results from the statewide provider survey to develop a web-based at-risk prevention toolkit comprising program modules, educational resources, and outreach materials that will be available to schools, professionals, and families throughout the state. The organization also holds an annual conference, which includes professional training opportunities in specific areas related to prevention of youth risk behavior, and provides regional trainings in local communities throughout the year.

Training of various stakeholders in prevention of youth risk behavior should include information regarding effective programming and best practices. As summarized in Rishel et al. (2007), multiple reviews have identified common characteristics of effective youth risk behavior prevention programs that cut across areas of risky sexual behavior, substance abuse, juvenile delinquency, and academic problems (Kirby, 1997, 2001; Morrissey et al., 1997; Nation et al., 2003; Weissberg, Kumpfer, & Seligman, 2003). The common characteristics are that the program is comprehensive, theoretically based, with sufficient dosing, appropriately timed, culturally relevant, utilizing interactive teaching methods, a well-trained staff, and evaluation.

Comprehensive. Comprehensive programs focus on the individual and the surrounding environment. They include multiple interventions aimed at affecting the target behavior and implement interventions in multiple settings. For example, programs aimed at reducing youth risk behavior should address risk and protective factors in all settings that directly impact youth, including the community, school, peer group, and family (Morrissey et al., 1997; Nation et al., 2003; Weissberg et al., 2003).

Theoretically based. Effective programs are based on a clear theoretical model that explains why the intervention should impact the target problem (Morrissey et al., 1997; Nation et al., 2003). Furthermore, implementation of the intervention is based on theoretical approaches that have demonstrated effectiveness at affecting other health-related behaviors (Kirby, 2001).

Sufficient dosage. Prevention programs must last a sufficient length of time and include enough contact hours of intervention to achieve the desired effect (Mulvey, Arthur, & Reppucci, 1993).

Appropriately timed. Effective programs are appropriately matched to the developmental stage of participants and are timed to occur prior to the onset or development of the problem behavior, usually focusing on antecedents or risk factors of the target problem (Weissberg et al., 2003).

Culturally relevant. Teaching methods and materials used in effective prevention programs must be culturally relevant to the target population. Materials and methods may need to be adapted to best apply to different cultural groups (Kirby, 1997; Weissberg et al., 2003). For example, previous research has demonstrated that many people living in rural communities strongly value family and community ties (Ali & McWhirter, 2006). These values need to be considered when implementing youth risk prevention programming in rural communities.

Interactive teaching methods. Effective programs utilize interactive teaching methods to involve participants and help them to personalize the information (Kirby, 2001; Tobler & Stratton, 1997), often including hands-on experiences that focus on skill development (Morrissey et al., 1997; Nation et al., 2003).

Well-trained staff. Well-trained staff are a critical component of effective programs. Staff chosen to implement the program must believe in the program and receive sufficient training to deliver the program well (Kirby, 1997, 2001; Weissberg et al., 2003).

Outcome evaluation or follow-up. Successful prevention programs include outcome evaluation or follow-up assessments to determine the long-term effects of the intervention (Morrissey et al., 1997; Nation et al., 2003).

DEVELOP COLLABORATIVE COMMUNITY PREVENTION PLANS

The above strategies are best implemented within a collaborative community prevention plan. Results from the statewide provider survey indicate that professionals who work with youth perceive that better collaboration and information sharing among community agencies is critical to effective prevention of adolescent risk behavior. This perception is supported by research that suggests that community-wide risk reduction is an effective approach to preventing youth risk behavior (Hawkins et al., 2002). Two specific models for developing and implementing community-based prevention plans that have been shown to be appropriate, effective, and feasible for rural communities include Communities that Care (CTC) and PROmoting School-community-university Partnerships to Enhance Resilience (PROSPER). The CTC model is a manualized program that mobilizes community members to identify specific risk and protective factors related to youth risk behavior in their community and then develop a comprehensive prevention plan (Hawkins et al., 2002). The PROSPER approach, supported by decades of National Institutes of Health–funded research (Spoth, 2007), facilitates the delivery of evidence-based prevention programs with youth and families by creating partnerships among Cooperative Extension programs located within land-grant universities, local schools, community members, and university-based researchers (Spoth, Greenberg, Bierman, & Redmond, 2004). It is important to note that CTC and PROSPER emphasize local community involvement and the formation of a community coalition of key stakeholders. This community-based approach fosters a sense of "ownership" of the resulting community-wide prevention plan, a critically important element of successful prevention efforts in the rural context. More information about CTC and PROSPER can be found at www.communitiesthatcare.net and www.prosper.ppsi.iastate.edu.

Limitations of the Study

Several limitations of this study should be noted. As noted in previous work, based on the adolescent and parent sample used in this study (Rishel et al., 2010), unique sample characteristics need to be considered. Adolescents and their parents chose whether to participate in the study after reviewing a brief project description, possibly resulting in selection bias. It is not possible to know if the results are generalizable to adolescents who would not have chosen to participate. In addition, most of the participants in the parent–adolescent study were female, despite the approximately equal representation of male and female adolescents in the classrooms and schools from which the sample was recruited. Either parent was invited to participate along with his or her child in the study. The consenting sample, however, consisted of mostly adolescent females and their mothers. Based on this sample characteristic and the fact that participants were all from the state of West Virginia, these findings may not be generalizable to other groups of adolescents. It is important to note, however, that descriptive analyses of main study variables revealed no significant differences based on gender, and controlling for gender in multivariate analyses did not affect the results. Similarly to the parent–adolescent study, all provider participants were from the state of West Virginia. In addition, providers chose to participate after receiving a request to complete the web-based survey through Survey Monkey. It is not possible to know if provider results are generalizable to providers who chose not to participate or providers located in other states. However, common challenges related to service provision in rural contexts suggest that provider perceptions in other rural areas may be similar.

CONCLUSION

Although mainly exploratory in nature, it is hoped that results from this study will inform the development and implementation of contextually appropriate prevention interventions in rural communities. Rural providers in this sample report belief that prevention of adolescent risk behavior is possible and express willingness to coordinate programming and share information among agencies to improve prevention interventions in their communities. This offers much hope for the future and points to the importance of developing community-wide prevention plans in rural areas.

REFERENCES

Ali, S. R., & McWhirter, S. R. (2006). Rural Appalachian youth's vocational/educational postsecondary aspirations. *Journal of Career Development, 33*, 87–111.

Atav, S., & Spencer, G. A. (2002). Health risk behaviors among adolescents attending rural, suburban, and urban schools: A comparative study. *Family and Community Health*, *25*, 53–64.

Centers for Disease Control & Prevention. (2009). *West Virginia 2009 and United States 2009 results*. Retrieved from www.cdc.gov/yrbss

Chilenski, S. M., & Greenberg, M. T. (2009). The importance of the community context in the epidemiology of early adolescent substance use and delinquency in a rural sample. *American Journal of Community Psychology*, *44*, 287–301.

Cottrell, S. A., Branstetter, S., Cottrell, L., Harris, C. V., Rishel, C. W., & Stanton, B. (2007). Development and validation of a parental monitoring instrument: Measuring how parents monitor adolescents' activities and risk behaviors. *Family Journal: Counseling and Therapy for Couples and Families*, *15*, 328–335.

Diaz, S. A., Secades-Villa, R., Errasti Perez, J. M., Fernandez-Hermida, J. R., Garcia-Rodriguez, O., & Carballo Crespo, J. L. (2006). Family predictors of parent participation in an adolescent drug abuse prevention program. *Drug and Alcohol Review*, *25*(4), 327–331.

Dunn, M. S., Ilapogu, V., Taylor, L., Naney, C., Blackwell, R., Wilder, R., & Givens, C. (2008). Self-reported substance use and sexual behaviors among adolescents in a rural state. *Journal of School Health*, *78*, 587–593.

Durlak, J. A. (1998). Common risk and protective factors in successful prevention programs. *American Journal of Orthopsychiatry*, *68*, 512–520.

Eber, L., Hyde, K., & Suter, J. C. (2011). Integrating wraparound into a schoolwide system of positive behavior supports. *Journal of Child and Family Studies*, *20*, 782–790.

Economic Research Service. (2012). *West Virginia state fact sheet*. Retrieved from http://www.ers.usda.gov/StateFacts/HTML2PDF/WV-Fact-Sheet.pdf

Francis, S. A. (2011). Using a framework to explore associations between parental substance use and the health outcomes of their adolescent children. *Journal of Child and Adolescent Substance Abuse*, *20*, 1–14.

Garmezy, N. (1985). Stress resilient children: The search for protective factors. In J. E. Stevenson (Ed.), *Recent research in developmental psychology: Journal of child psychology and psychiatry book* (pp. 213–233). Oxford, England: Pergamon.

Greenberger, E., Chen, C., & Beam, M. R. (1998). The role of "very important" nonparental adults in adolescent development. *Journal of Youth and Adolescence*, *27*, 321–343.

Guilamo-Ramos, V., Jaccard, J., Dittus, P., & Bouris, A. (2006). Parental expertise, trustworthiness, and accessibility: Parent-adolescent communication and adolescent risk behavior. *Journal of Marriage and Family*, *68*, 1229–1246.

Hawkins, D. J., Catalano, R. F., & Arthur, M. W. (2002). Promoting science-based prevention in communities. *Addictive Behaviors*, *27*, 951–976.

Hawkins, D. J., Catalano, R. F., & Miller, J. Y. (1992). Risk and protective factors for alcohol and other drug problems in adolescent and early adulthood: Implications for substance abuse prevention. *Psychological Bulletin*, *112*, 64–105.

Howard, D., Qiu, Y., & Boekeloo, B. (2003). Personal and social contextual correlates of adolescent dating violence. *Journal of Adolescent Health*, *33*, 9–17.

Ice, C., & Cottrell, L. (2010, April). *Good parenting: Exploring home- and public-schooled adolescent perceptions of their risk behaviors and their parent's good parenting behaviors.* Poster presented at the Conference of Human Development, New York, NY.

Kafka, R., & London, P. (1991). Communication in relationships and adolescent substance use: The influence of parents and friends. *Adolescence, 26,* 587–598.

Kapadia, F., Frye, V., Bonner, S., Emmanuel, P. J., Samples, C. L., & Latka, M. H. (2012). Perceived peer safer sex norms and sexual risk behaviors among substance-using Latino adolescents. *AIDS Education and Prevention, 24,* 27–40.

King, K. M., & Chassin, L. (2004). Mediating and moderated effects of adolescent behavioral undercontrol and parenting: The prediction of drug use disorders in emerging adulthood. *Psychology of Addictive Behaviors, 18,* 26–43.

Kirby, D. (1997). *No easy answers: Research findings on programs to reduce teen pregnancy.* Washington, DC: National Campaign to Prevent Teen Pregnancy.

Kirby, D. (2001). *Emerging answers: Research findings on programs to reduce teen pregnancy.* Washington, DC: National Campaign to Prevent Teen Pregnancy.

Kolbe, L. J., Kann, L., & Collins, J. (1993). The youth risk behavior surveillance system: overview of the youth risk behavior surveillance system. *Public Health Reports, 106,* 1–9.

Kumpfer, K. L., Alvarado, R., Smith, P., & Bellamny, N. (2002). Cultural sensitivity in universal family-based prevention interventions. *Prevention Science, 3,* 241–244.

Kumpfer, K. L., Alvarado, R., Tait, C., & Turner, C. (2002). Effectiveness of school-based family and children's skills training for substance abuse prevention among 6–8 year old rural children. *Psychology of Addictive Behaviors, 16,* 65–71.

Kumpfer, K. L., Alvarado, R., & Whiteside, H. O. (2003). Family-based interventions for substance use and misuse prevention. *Substance Use and Misuse, 38,* 1759–1787.

Li, X., Feigelman, S., & Stanton, B. F. (2000). Perceived parental monitoring and health risk behaviors among urban low-income African-American children and adolescents. *Journal of Adolescent Health, 27,* 43–48.

Merikangas, K. R., Dierker, L. C., & Szatmari, P. (1998). Children of parents with substance abuse disorders had higher rates of conduct disorder and substance use. *Journal of Child Psychology and Psychiatry, 39,* 711–720.

Miller, C. H., Burgoon, M., Grandpre, J. R., & Alvaro, E. M. (2006). Identifying principal risk factors for the initiation of adolescent smoking behaviors: The significance of psychological reactance. *Health Communication, 19,* 241–252.

Morrissey, E., Wandersman, A., Seybolt, D., Nation, M., Crusto, C., & Davino, K. (1997). Toward a framework for bridging the gap between science and practice in prevention: A focus on evaluator and practitioner perspectives. *Evaluation and Program Planning, 20,* 367–377.

Mulvey, E., Arthur, M., & Reppucci, D. (1993). The prevention and treatment of juvenile delinquency: A review of the research. *Clinical Psychology Review, 13,* 133–167.

Nation, M., Crusto, C., Wandersman, A., Kumpfer, K. L., Seybolt, D., Morrissey-Kane, E., & Davino, K. (2003). What works in prevention: Principles of effective prevention programs. *American Psychologist, 58,* 449–456.

Puskar, K. R., Tusaie-Mumford, K., Sereika, S., & Lamb, J. (1999). Health concerns and risk behaviors of rural adolescents. *Journal of Community Health Nursing, 16,* 109–119.

Rai, A. A., Stanton, B. F., Wu, Y., Li, X., Galbraith, J., Cottrell, L., ... Burns, J. (2003). Relative influences of perceived parental monitoring and perceived peer involvement on adolescent risk behaviors: An analysis of six cross-sectional data sets. *Journal of Adolescent Health*, *33*, 108–118.

Rishel, C. W., Cottrell, L., Cottrell, S. A., Stanton, B. F., Gibson, C. A., & Bougher, K. (2007). Exploring adolescents' relationships with non-parental adults using the Non-Parental Adult Inventory (N.P.A.I.). *Child and Adolescent Social Work Journal*, *24*, 495–508.

Rishel, C. W., Cottrell, L., Stanton, B., Cottrell, S., & Branstetter, S. (2010). The buffering effect of non-parental adults in the relationship between parent-adolescent communication and adolescent risk behavior. *Families in Society*, *91*, 371–377.

Rishel, C. W., Sales, E., & Koeske, G. F. (2005). Relationships with non-parental adults and child behavior. *Child and Adolescent Social Work Journal*, *22*, 19–34.

Smith, C., & Carlson, B. E. (1997). Stress, coping, and resilience in children and youth. *Social Service Review*, *72*, 231–256.

Song, E., Smiler, A. P., Wagoner, K. G., Wolfson, M. (2012). Everyone says it's OK: Adolescents' perceptions of peer, parent, and community alcohol norms, alcohol consumption, and alcohol-related consequences. *Substance Use and Misuse*, *47*, 86–98.

Spoth, R. (2007). Opportunities to meet challenges in rural prevention research: Findings from an evolving community-university partnership model. *Journal of Rural Health*, *23*, 42–54.

Spoth, R., Greenberg, M., Bierman, K., & Redmond, C. (2004). PROSPER community-university partnership model for public education systems: Capacity-building for evidence-based, competence-building prevention. *Prevention Science*, *5*, 31–39.

Spoth, R., Guyll, M., & Day, S. (2002). Universal family-focused interventions in alcohol-use disorder prevention: Cost-effectiveness and cost-benefit analyses of two interventions. *Journal of Studies on Alcohol*, *63*, 219–228.

Stanton, B. F., Li, X., Galbraith, J., Cornick, G., Feigelman, S., Kaljee, L., & Zhou, Y. (2000). Parental underestimates of adolescent risk behavior: A randomized, controlled trial of a parental monitoring intervention. *Journal of Adolescent Health*, *26*, 18–26.

Sugai, G., & Horner, R. H. (2008). What we know about preventing problem behavior in schools. *Exceptionality*, *16*, 67–77.

Sullivan, C. J., Childs, K. K., & O'Connell, D. (2010). Adolescent risk behavior subgroups: An empirical assessment. *Journal of Youth and Adolescence*, *39*, 541–562.

Tobler, N. S., & Stratton, H. H. (1997). Effectiveness of school-based drug prevention programs: A meta-analysis of the research. *Journal of Primary Prevention*, *18*, 71–128.

Weissberg, R. P., Kumpfer, K. L., & Seligman, M. E. P. (2003). Prevention that works for children and youth. *American Psychologist*, *58*, 425–432.

Werner, E. E. (1992). The children of Kauai: Resiliency and recovery in adolescence and adulthood. *Journal of Adolescent Health*, *13*, 262–268.

Werner, E. E. (1995). Resilience in development. *Current Directions in Psychological Science*, *4*, 81–85.

Wu, Y., Stanton, B. F., Galbraith, J., Kaljee, L., Cottrell, L., Li, X., & Harris, C. V. (2003). Sustaining and broadening intervention impact: A longitudinal randomized trial of three adolescent risk reduction approaches. *Pediatrics*, *111*, 32–38.

Rural Women's Transitions to Motherhood: Understanding Social Support in a Rural Community

CHRISTOPHER D. GJESFJELD

University of North Dakota, Grand Forks, North Dakota

ADDIE WEAVER

University of Michigan, Ann Arbor, Michigan

KATHRYN SCHOMMER

The Village Family Service Center, Fargo, North Dakota

Social support protects women from various negative consequences, yet we have little understanding of how rural women acquire and utilize social support. Using interviews of 24 women in a North Dakota community, this research sought to understand how rural women were supported as new mothers. One, familial women and partners were vital supports to these women. Two, medical professionals were expected to provide only the "medical part," consisting of medical information and delivery procedures. Finally, dangers of limited social support were examined. Peer support programs and screening are discussed as potential avenues for addressing maternal distress in rural communities.

Rural women's health is a relatively new area of scholarship that considers the interrelated aspects of physical and mental health (Thorndyke, 2005). The psychological well-being of women transitioning to motherhood in rural communities has a significant impact on their prenatal, delivery, and postpartum experiences and should be of great concern for health professionals aiding women in these contexts. A number of issues can complicate women's mental health and the health of their children, including postpartum depression, family conflict, economic stress, and maternal and/or familial substance abuse (Silver, Heneghan, Bauman, & Stein, 2006). Addressing these issues in rural communities can be problematic given the limited accessibility and availability of providers, as well as rural beliefs regarding help seeking (Fox, Merwin, & Blank, 1995; New Freedom Commission on Mental Health, 2004). Because many rural women do not readily utilize formal service providers (e.g., social workers, psychologists, doulas) during their transition to motherhood, it is imperative to understand how rural women receive support in their informal social networks. Our research explores how rural women seek and receive formal and informal support during their pregnancies and after the birth of their children. Understanding women's methods for seeking and receiving social support will aid women's health providers and researchers in developing a more nuanced understanding of how social support is utilized by rural women.

POSTPARTUM DEPRESSION AND MATERNAL DISTRESS

Depression is the most commonly identified risk factor for postpartum women. Roughly 7% of women experience a major depressive episode at some point in the 3-month period following the birth of their child (see review by O'Hara, 2009). When untreated, postpartum depression has a dramatic impact on the quality of life of mothers and appears to negatively affect parenting (Downey & Coyne, 1990; Goodman, 2007). In addition, nondepressed mothers can have postpartum experiences that are equally distressing but do not fit neatly into a purely psychiatric framework (Mauthner, 1999).

In contrast to the terminology of postpartum depression, which Barclay and Lloyd (1996) argued accuses women of their own distress, the concept of "maternal distress" is conceptualized as an experience that includes the social and familial connections that are fundamentally linked to one's psychological health (Barclay & Lloyd, 1996). These social connections, or "connecting responses," coined by Emmanuel and St. John (2010), are the social, familial, and community connections that are vital determinants for how an individual will cope with stress and adjustment. For many women, the support received from close family members and friends is intimately connected to their adjustment as mothers. Emmanuel and St. John (2010) claimed that without these connecting responses, a woman "does not feel accepted, loved, needed and respected, whilst a lack of tangible goods and services can make a woman feel instrumentally disconnected" (p. 2111). These resources, emotional and practical, are critical to the emotional health of women transitioning to motherhood.

CONNECTING RESPONSES AND SOCIAL SUPPORT

These connecting responses that Emmanuel and John (2010) saw as a vital component of maternal distress confirm a significant finding in the empirical research on women's mental health; social support and social networks protect pregnant and postpartum women from psychological distress (Boyce & Hickey, 2005; Collins, Dunkel-Schetter, Lobel, & Scrimshaw, 1993; Hopkins & Campbell, 2008; Zachariah, 2004). Generally speaking, social support can be defined as a "social fund from which people may draw when handling stressors" (Thoits, 1995, p. 64). The concept of social support is typically operationalized as functional or perceived support that measures the extent to which an individual believes that he or she will be assisted in a particular way (e.g., emotional support, tangible support, such as money or childcare assistance, informational support). Of particular note, the social support of one's partner during pregnancy appears particularly important in reducing distress (Kearns, Neuwelt, Hitchman, & Lennan, 1997). For example, in a study of 129 low-income, primarily Latina women, the satisfaction with partner support was shown to be associated with improved labor progress, higher Apgar scores among infants, and less depression in the postpartum period among women.

Qualitative accounts of women's transition to motherhood in three English speaking countries have also provided clues as to the linkages between limited social support and maternal distress. For example, 55 first-time mothers in Australia who perceived a lack of emotional support and practical assistance from either their partners or other women reported a sense of "feeling alone" (Barclay, Everitt, Rogan, Schmied, & Wyllie, 1997). In Mauthner's (1999) qualitative analysis of 18 Canadian women with postpartum depression, mothers frequently felt that their inability to share their emotional state with others and the concern that others would not be receptive to their experiences contributed to their emotional distress. In addition, Raymond (2009) found that poor partner support encouraged women to "go inside" and not express their anxieties, a process known as "self-silencing." The inability to share these anxieties became associated with feelings of isolation and loneliness. These qualitative accounts point to the interconnected experience of maternal distress and poor social support for mothers of infants.

Quantitative and qualitative research demonstrates that social support is vital to positive emotional outcomes for women transitioning to motherhood, yet very limited work explores rural women's experiences receiving and accepting social support. It is critical to understand rural women's social support experiences to identify how this resource is acquired. Ultimately, a better understanding of how rural women in transition to motherhood access social support in their community can aid rural providers and researchers in providing services that better meet their needs.

RURAL WOMEN AND SOCIAL SUPPORT: THE RURAL CONTEXT

Despite the varying roles for social workers in rural settings, formal supports are often limited in rural America. The majority of counties designated as

Health Professional Shortage Areas are also in rural communities (Bird, Dempsey, & Hartley, 2001; Gamm, Stone, & Pittman, 2003; Mulder et al., 2000). According to Fordyce, Chen, Doescher, and Hart (2007), rural areas in the United States account for 19.2% of the population, yet only have 11.4% of physicians. More specifically to physicians specializing in obstetrics or gynecology, urban areas maintain 12.8 physicians for every 100,000 people whereas small, rural and isolated small, rural communities have 4.8 and 1.5 physicians per 100,000, respectively. The consequence is that rural women need to travel greater distances for care and their choice of providers is more limited (Gjesfjeld & Jung, 2011).

Rural women have also essentially been denied equal access to mental health care, given its limited availability in rural America (Letvak, 2002; McCabe & Macnee, 2002). Rural and urban residents have similar rates of psychological distress (Hauenstein et al., 2006; Kessler et al., 1994; Robins & Regier, 1991), yet 75% of rural counties lack a psychiatrist (Holzer, Goldsmith, & Ciarlo, 1998). Although urban counties, on average, report an excess of 13 specialty mental health organizations, rural counties average fewer than two (Goldsmith, Wagenfeld, Manderscheid, & Stiles, 1997).

Even when providers are available, rural residents tend to exhibit a preference for informal support networks, often seeking help, advice, and information from friends and family rather than contacting formal providers (Fox, Blank, Rovnyak, & Barnett, 2001; Fox et al., 1995; Young, Giles, & Plantz, 1982). Literature suggests that health beliefs and stigma are common in rural communities and contribute to the preference for informal support (Hill & Fraser, 1995; Letvak, 2002; Rost, Smith, & Taylor, 1993; Stamm, 2003). Gaining access to appropriate health and mental health treatment for people living in rural areas involves substantial transportation barriers, including distance-related travel burden, lack of public transportation, and weather (Fortney, Rost, Zhang, & Warren, 1999; Fox et al., 2001). Furthermore, cost presents a considerable deterrent to obtaining services for rural Americans who are more likely to live in poverty, more likely to be uninsured or underinsured, and less likely to qualify for Medicaid than urban Americans (Beck, Jijon, & Edwards, 1996; Human & Wasem, 1991; Mueller, Patil, & Ulrich, 1997; Mulder et al., 2000).

Culture, or a set of beliefs, norms, values, and traditions shared by a group of people, can have a strong influence on treatment-seeking behaviors. Rural persons' health beliefs, including a cultural emphasis on self-reliance and independence, can have an important impact on health care decisions related to mental health care (Hill & Fraser, 1995; Letvak, 2002; Rost et al., 1993). Health beliefs commonly endorsed in rural areas support the role performance model of health, which assumes health as long as one is able to be productive, work, and carry out usual role functions (Weinert & Long, 1990). This belief system supports seeking medical attention only when problems are severe, and it likely contributes to the devaluation and subsequent underutilization of health care services. Further, cultural values held by rural Americans, such as self-reliance and independence, often lead to the belief that mental health concerns are a personal weakness rather than a medical illness (Rost, Fortney, Fisher, & Smith, 2002). This view of mental illness contributes to high levels of shame and stigma around mental health treatment in rural areas (Stamm, 2003). As a result of these health beliefs, some have argued that rural populations adopt unique culturally endorsed coping strategies based on traditional self-care and the support of informal networks (Fox et al., 1995; Young et al., 1982).

PURPOSE OF THE RESEARCH

Given the critical transition to motherhood for women and the documented research demonstrating the significant contribution of social support, it is important that health professionals are aware of how rural mothers acquire and utilize social support in their social network. As we considered the rural context and social support literature, three key questions guided our research. Although these questions were not asked verbatim to the mothers, these three questions suggest the initial spirit of inquiry.

1. Who do rural mothers rely upon in their informal network?
2. What types of support do they receive from their formal network, specifically medical professionals, during pregnancy, birth, and the postpartum period?
3. How is social support connected to their maternal distress?

METHOD

Participants and Setting

This work reports findings from semistructured, in-depth, qualitative interviews conducted in November and December of 2010 with 24 "new" mothers (i.e., mothers with a child younger than age 18 months) receiving services through the Special Supplemental Nutrition Program for Women, Infants, and Children (WIC) in a rural county in North Dakota. To be eligible for this program that provides nutrition education to low-income women, families must have household incomes that do not exceed 185% of the federal poverty line. These women were, on average, age 24 with an age range between 18 and 32. Seventeen mothers (71%) were White, six mother (25%) were Hispanic, and one mother (4%) was Native American. Fifteen (63%) of the mothers were married, and nine (38%) were single. In terms of employment status, nine (38%) mothers stated that they were "stay at home moms," 13 (54%) were working either part-time or full-time, and two (8%) noted that they were students. On average, mothers had travelled 50 miles one way to a community of 60,000 that had maternity services during their third trimester and for the actual delivery services.

Data Collection

Semistructured, in-depth interviews explored women's perceptions of their transition from pregnancy to the current day. The overarching goal of this project was to identify, from the rural mothers' point of view, factors affecting women's transition to motherhood, with special attention given to learning about social supports received from formal and informal networks. Interviews were scheduled in conjunction with the women's regular scheduled appointments. Interviews were digitally recorded and transcribed verbatim. A female research assistant who had finished her course work for the masters in social work degree conducted all interviews. The University of North Dakota's Institutional Review Board approved procedures for the study. Over the course of data collection, the principal investigator and the interviewer met regularly to ensure comparable questions were being utilized in the interviews while maintaining flexibility, which allowed new information to be identified and incorporated.

Data Analysis

Thematic analysis was utilized to analyze the qualitative data after the digital recordings were transcribed and checked for accuracy. The analysis began with in vivo or line-by-line coding, an open coding strategy that focuses on minute aspects of the data and categorizes responses with participants' own language and meanings whenever possible (Strauss & Corbin, 1990). This led to the development of thematic categories representing common themes that had emerged. The in vivo coding and thematic categories that we identified were discussed in meetings between the principal investigator and the graduate student. If both of us confirmed that a particular theme was present, we further collapsed these themes into core categories that represented the most variation in mothers' perceptions and behavior (Strauss, 1987). The principal investigator and interviewer engaged in ongoing dialogue over multiple months to connect the line-by-line coding to broader themes and interpret the emerging categories. This coding and interpretation process produced a comprehensive inventory of important ideas, expressions, terms, and phrases that reflects the language and views of participants and best exemplifies the core thematic categories. Quantifying techniques (e.g., tables) were also developed to confirm consensus around these broader themes across the 24 interviews. Our analysis yielded three core categories relevant to understanding the role of social support during rural women's transition to motherhood: (1) other women and partners as vital social supports, (2) informational support from formal supports, and (3) the potential consequences of limited social support.

FINDINGS

"Just There for Me": Women and Partners as Vital Social Support

When we inquired about who was supportive in the respondents' lives, the most common answer was other women in their family (e.g., mothers, mother-in-laws, sisters). Other women, particularly those that were mothers, were able to provide a context of having "been there," which many women perceived as emotionally stabilizing. Familial women offered the mothers a place to emotionally express their joys and trials during the transition from pregnancy to having an infant, "[My mom] Listen[ed] to me talk . . . 'cause it was just me and [my two children] and there was no dad around." Another mother's reaction provided a visual symbol that represented the important bond with family, "My sister. She stayed with me the whole time. They [the hospital] even gave her a nightgown to sleep with me. She slept in the next bed." This emotional space with other women in the family also opened up opportunities for women to ask questions that probed their own fears and anxieties. For example, one woman described how her mother provided guidance:

> The pain, the confusion, the crying, she was there. I would call her and say, "mom, I don't get this, why is this happening?" She would say, "you are pregnant; this is going to happen, and this is going to happen."

Beside merely "being there," these mothers also voiced that practical assistance was particularly helpful in the postpartum period. For example, some women had cesarean section (C-section) births. Women commented on how they were helped after recovering from their C-section, "My mom stayed a week and kinda helped me, you know, 'cause I have a two-level apartment . . . 'cause it was kinda hard with my C-section to go up and down the stairs. " Another mother made a similar remark:

> She came and stayed with us . . . [and] I didn't have to do much, you know, just laying around and she took care of the baby for a couple days and I just got to sit there and she did everything.

In sum, women in the family were vital and offered emotional and practical support to the mothers we interviewed. Familial women normalized any anxieties mothers had during pregnancy, delivery, and the postpartum period and offered them practical assistance when needed.

Without exception, the mothers talked of familial women who were in geographic proximity to them. Talking to women on the phone, sending and receiving e-mail, or through video-conference technologies (e.g., Skype) were rarely discussed. However, two mothers mentioned that they used Facebook updates to communicate the delivery to family and friends in their community.

In addition to familial women, intimate partners were also important. Support from partners seemed to focus on providing physical comfort to women during pregnancy as well as practical assistance with household tasks in the postpartum period. This mother communicates how her partner helped her during pregnancy, "He was rubbing my feet and he'd give me back rubs and made sure I always got whatever I was craving." Although this type of support from intimate partners appeared fairly common during pregnancy, the partners appeared engaged in different tasks, such as assisting in feedings and general housework, after the birth of the baby. This mother comments on one task in which her partner engaged, "My dad helped my boyfriend finish setting up the crib because there was like one piece that would not screw in there or something because the hole was too small so he helped him set up the crib."

Another mother commented on how her partner helped with their new infant:

> And he would, you know, change her and he would give her to me and get the bottles ready and, you know, put her outfits on her and stuff like that. I mean, he was, from day one, very helpful.

Professional Supports: Pamphlets, Pamphlets, Pamphlets!

When asked about their expectations of maternity care and delivery, few women expressed explicit expectations of the medical professionals that they encountered (i.e., physicians, nurses). They desired the medical professionals to do the "medical part" and didn't seem to desire or expect emotional support from their providers. The resources provided to pregnant and new mothers were provided in a didactic method emphasizing books, pamphlets, and videos, or as one mother commented, "[you] watch a whole bunch of videos." In nearly every interview, new mothers said that questions about their new infant would be answered by their family. Professional supports clearly were seen in a different light and offered a specific focus. These quotes depict what the women in the study received from health professionals, "[They provided me with a] whole book-type deal...they told me to read it and it would tell me what I need to know." In this interview, the mother seemed to suggest that prenatal care could offer a more enhanced or personal experience:

> They both had a big bag of brochures and different resources...so I did have brochures and I did have a book that I read...but I would have rather had the prenatal care but I just could not afford it at the time.

In these interviews, when asked about the maternity care received, most women indicated that they were satisfied with their interactions with medical professionals. In rare cases when dissatisfaction was voiced, women would generally rationalize why the care may not have been optimal and did not believe the provider was to blame. One respondent expressed how she felt after she realized the female provider who was to deliver her baby was on vacation, "I was kinda disappointed but I understand that she can't be there every single time or she would never have a personal life, I guess." It became clear that women viewed supports from health care providers in a very focused way, "They monitor and deliver my baby."

These providers also provided a plethora of pamphlets, yet it was unclear as to how helpful the women found this information. These women did not seem to receive emotional support from medical professionals nor did they generally expect it to be provided.

Are Rural Women at Risk for Maternal Distress?

The majority of these rural women expressed satisfaction with the social support they received from others. They described receiving emotional and tangible support from their families, as well as informational support from medical providers about their pregnancy and newborns. Despite their low socioeconomic status, the 24 women interviewed appear fairly resilient in the face of the stressors of new motherhood. They maintain strong familial ties that help them in practical and emotional ways.

The question remains, however, which rural mothers are at risk for maternal distress? Consistent with our finding that emotional support was an integral aspect of the experience for rural women, those without family supports seem to be at particular risk of loneliness, isolation, and depression during and after their pregnancies. Three of these mothers described limited social support from others and expressed specific concerns related to this lack of a social support network. These mothers had few extended family members or other ties to the community. One specific interview exemplifies this theme and some of the potential consequences, "Being a first-time mom was really hard; really, really hard for me. I have no family here; I only have his [husband's family] here and they were not really helpful so I had to do it by myself basically."

In another part of the interview, this woman specifically mentioned the formal supports of the WIC office as helpful for her. In her interview, she was one of the few women that also talked about experiencing the "baby blues,":

> For a while there after I had my baby, I had the baby blues. So like I did not want to do anything. Then I didn't know how to make her stop crying. It was really hard . . . I would cry for no reason after I had my first one because I was lost. I didn't go out of my house.

Given the geographic isolation from professional services coupled with the lack of family social support, we were concerned by interviews such as this. If medical professionals are unable to detect postpartum depression and women have few supports, they appear to be particularly vulnerable to the negative impact of depression.

DISCUSSION AND IMPLICATIONS

New mothers in our research were highly engaged with other women within their own family of origin and appeared to use these networks as sources of emotional and tangible support over the course of their pregnancy and in the post-partum period. The women in their families seemed to provide different types of assistance to these "new" mothers: advice on childrearing, assistance in occasional childcare, and practical assistance with household tasks and chores. Partners, when present, also offered assistance. Respondents seemed to suggest that this assistance was more practical (e.g., change the baby, put together the crib, do laundry) and less emotional than support from other women.

When family support was present, it appeared to be a protective factor providing strength and additional resources to rural women. Others have identified the reliance of rural populations on informal supports. For rural women transitioning to motherhood, the support received from familial women and partners was an important and consistent finding in our interviews. Unfortunately, relying solely on support from family may be problematic if a woman has family relationships that are wrought with conflict or are not present. As Rook (1984) noted in her work on social support, conflict in social networks can have serious negative effects on one's emotional health.

Given the importance of social support to rural women in this study, as well as other qualitative and quantitative connections between social support and mental health outcomes, we suggest that social workers in hospital and community settings better assess the quality of women's social supports. Just as routine use of screening tools for depression can open doors to treatment, assessment of social support can be the first step in understanding sources of risk and resiliency in the social networks of a rural mother (Ervins, Theofrastous, & Galvin, 2000). For example, medical professionals could make one simple observation: Is anyone with this woman during her delivery? If the woman feels or appears minimally supported, this information may be helpful for the social worker or other health professionals in terms of determining necessary resources.

Besides this research pointing to the important emphasis rural women place on familial support, this research also provides interesting insights into how rural women and medical providers engage with one another. When we asked these women to reflect on their interactions with health professionals, the assistance they received was informational (e.g., pamphlets, videos, books) and specific to the skills associated with the delivery. Despite these women's positive impressions about their health care experiences, we feel that these women's experiences illuminate some opportunities in which health professionals, in the hospital and in the community, could be increasingly relevant to the emotional adjustment of these women.

In terms of implications for practice, we recommend a mentorship or "buddy-type" model for aiding mothers with little support. Given the particular helpfulness women felt from older women in their families, it is conceivable that a mentor may replicate a similar family function that our interviewees identified. Social workers are well prepared to facilitate development of such programs in rural communities (see manymothers.org for specific strategies for developing a volunteer service for families with newborns).

Families play a vital role for rural mothers with infants. Social work professionals should assert their expertise in medical settings and communities so rural mothers are provided with the social support they require during this important transition. Although the specific needs of mothers will vary, social work professionals can work to assess the social support network of new mothers, assist our medical professionals in being more emotionally responsive to the needs of new mothers, and remind policy stakeholders of the access challenges specific to the rural experience.

REFERENCES

Barclay, L., Everitt, L., Rogan, F., Schmied, V., & Wyllie, A. (1997). Becoming a mother—An analysis of women's experience of early motherhood. *Journal of Advanced Nursing, 25*, 719–728.

Barclay, L. M., & Lloyd, B. (1996). The misery of motherhood: Alternative approaches to maternal distress. *Midwifery, 12*, 136–139.

Beck, R. W., Jijon, C. R., & Edwards, J. B. (1996). The relationships among gender, perceived financial barriers to care, and health status in a rural population. *Journal of Rural Health, 12*, 188–196.

Bird, D. C., Dempsey, P., & Hartley, D. (2001). *Addressing mental health workforce needs in underserved rural areas: Accomplishments and challenges (Working Paper #23)*. Portland: Maine Rural Health Research Center, Institute for Health Policy, Edmund S. Muskie School of Public Service, University of Southern Maine.

Boyce, P., & Hickey, A. (2005). Psychosocial risk factors to major depression after childbirth. *Social Psychiatry and Psychiatric Epidemiology, 40*, 605–612.

Collins, N. L., Dunkel-Schetter, C., Lobel, M., & Scrimshaw, S. C. M. (1993). Social support in pregnancy: Psychosocial correlates of birth outcomes and postpartum depression. *Journal of Personality and Social Psychology, 65*(6), 1243–1258.

Downey, G., & Coyne, J. C. (1990). Children of depressed parents: An integrative review. *Psychological Bulletin, 108*(1), 50–76.

Emmanuel, E., & St. John, W. (2010). Maternal distress: A concept analysis. *Journal of Advanced Nursing, 66*(9), 2104–2115.

Ervins, G. G., Theofrastous, J. P., & Galvin, S. L. (2000). Postpartum depression: A comparison of screening and routine clinical evaluation. *American Journal of Obstetrics and Gynecology, 182*(5), 1080–1082.

Fordyce, M. A., Chen, F. M., Doescher, M. P., & Hart, G. (2007). *2005 physician supply and distribution in rural areas of the United States.* Seattle: WWAMI Rural Health Research Center, University of Washington.

Fortney, J., Rost, K., Zhang, M., & Warren, J. (1999). The impact of geographic accessibility on the intensity and quality of depression treatment. *Medical Care, 37,* 884–893.

Fox, J., Merwin, E., & Blank, M. (1995). De facto mental health services in the rural south. *Journal of Health Care for the Poor and Underserved, 6,* 434–468.

Fox, J. C., Blank, M., Rovnyak, V. G., & Barnett, R. Y. (2001). Barriers to help seeking for mental disorders in a rural impoverished population. *Community Mental Health Journal, 37,* 421–436.

Gamm, L. G., Stone, S., & Pittman, S. (2003). *Mental health and mental disorders—A rural challenge. Rural Healthy People 2010: A companion document to Health People 2010 (Vol. 1).* College Station: Southwest Rural Health Research Center, School of Rural Public Health, The Texas A&M University System Health Science Center.

Gjesfjeld, C. D., & Jung, J.-K. (2011). How far?: Using Geographical Information Systems (GIS) to examine maternity care access for expectant mothers in a rural state. *Social Work in Health Care, 50*(9), 682–693.

Goldsmith, H. F., Wagenfeld, M. O., Manderscheid, R. W., & Stiles, D. (1997). Specialty mental health services in metropolitan and nonmetropolitan areas: 1983 and 1990. *Administration & Policy in Mental Health, 24,* 475–488.

Goodman, S. H. (2007). Depression in mothers. *Annual Review of Clinical Psychology, 3,* 107–135.

Hauenstein, E. J., Petterson, S., Merwin, E., Rovnyak, V., Heise, B., & Wagner, D. (2006). Rurality, gender, and mental health treatment. *Family Community Health, 29,* 169–185.

Hill, C. E., & Fraser, G. J. (1995). Local knowledge and rural mental health reform. *Community Mental Health Journal, 31,* 553–568.

Holzer, C. E., Goldsmith, H. F., & Ciarlo, J. A. (1998). *Chapter 16: Effects of rural–urban county type on the availability of health and mental health care providers. Mental Health, United States (DHHS Pub. No. SMA99-3285).* Washington, DC: Superintendent of Documents, U.S. Government Printing Office.

Hopkins, J., & Campbell, S. B. (2008). Development and validation of a scale to assess social support in the postpartum period. *Archives of Women's Mental Health, 11,* 57–65.

Human, J., & Wasem, C. (1991). Rural mental health in America. *American Psychologist, 46,* 240–243.

Kearns, R. A., Neuwelt, P. M., Hitchman, B., & Lennan, M. (1997). Social support and psychological distress before and after childbirth. *Health and Social Care in the Community, 5*(5), 296–308.

Kessler, R. C., McGonagle, K. A., Zhao, S., Nelson, C. B., Hughes, M., Eshleman, S., . . . Kendler, K. S. (1994). Lifetime and 12-month prevalence of DSM-III-R psychiatric disorders in the United States: Results from the national comorbidity survey. *Archives of General Psychiatry, 51,* 8–19.

Letvak, S. (2002). The importance of social support for rural mental health. *Issues in Mental Health Nursing, 23*, 249–261.

Mauthner, N. S. (1999). "Feeling low and feeling really bad about feeling low": Women's experiences of motherhood and postpartum depression. *Canadian Psychology, 40*(2), 143–161.

McCabe, S., & Macnee, C. L. (2002). Weaving a new safety net of mental health care in rural America: A model of integrated practice. *Issues in Mental Health Nursing, 23*, 263–278.

Mueller, K., Patil, K., & Ulrich, F. (1997). Lengthening spells of uninsurance and their consequences. *Journal of Rural Health, 13*(1), 29–37.

Mulder, P. L., Kenkel, M., Shellenberger, S., Constantine, M. G., Streiegel, R., Sears, S. F., ... Hager, A. (2000). *The behavioral health care needs of rural women.* Washington, DC: Committee on Rural Health, American Psychological Association.

New Freedom Commission on Mental Health. (2004). *Subcommittee on rural issues: Background paper* (Pub. No. SMA-04-3890). Rockville, MD: U.S. Department of Health and Human Services.

O'Hara, M. W. (2009). Postpartum depression: What we know. *Journal of Clinical Psychology, 65*(12), 1258–1269.

Raymond, J. E. (2009). "Creating a safety net": Women's experiences of antenatal depression and their identification of helpful community support and services during pregnancy. *Midwifery, 25*, 39–49.

Robins, L. M., & Reiger, D. A. (Eds.). (1991). *Psychiatric disorders in America: The Epidemiological Catchment Area Study.* New York, NY: Free Press.

Rook, K. S. (1984). The negative side of social interaction: Impact on psychological well-being. *Journal of Personality and Social Psychology, 46*(5), 1097–1108.

Rost, K., Fortney, J., Fisher, E., & Smith, J. (2002). Use, quality, and outcomes of care for mental health: The rural perspective. *Medical Care Research and Review, 59*(3), 231–265.

Rost, K., Smith, G. R., & Taylor, J. L. (1993). Rural–urban differences in stigma and the use of care for depressive disorders. *Journal of Rural Health, 9*, 57–62.

Silver, E. J., Heneghan, A. M., Bauman, L. J., & Stein, R. E. K. (2006). The relationship of depressive symptoms to parenting competence and social support in inner-city mothers of young children. *Maternal and Child Health Journal, 10*, 105–112.

Stamm, B. H. (2003). *Rural behavioral health care: An interdisciplinary guide.* Washington, DC: American Psychological Association.

Strauss, A. L. (1987). *Qualitative analysis for social scientists.* New York, NY: Cambridge University Press.

Strauss, A. L., & Corbin, J. (1990). *Basics of qualitative research: Grounded theory procedures and techniques.* Newbury Park, CA: Sage.

Thoits, P. A. (1995). Stress, coping, and social support processes: Where are we? What next? *Journal of Health and Social Behavior, 35*(Extra Issue), 53–79.

Thorndyke, L. E. (2005). Rural women's health: A research agenda for the future. *Women's Health Issues, 15*, 200–203.

Weinert, C., & Long, K. (1990). Rural families and health care: Refining the knowledge base. In D. Unger & M. Sussman (Eds.), *Families in community settings: Interdisciplinary perspectives* (pp. 57–76). Binghamton, NY: Hawthorne.

Young, C. E., Giles, D. E., & Plantz, M. C. (1982). Natural networks: Help-giving and help-seeking in two rural communities. *American Journal of Community Psychology, 10*, 457–469.

Zachariah, R. (2004). Attachment, social support, life stress, and psychological well-being in pregnant low-income women: A pilot study. *Clinical Excellence for Nurse Practitioners, 8*(2), 60–67.

Influencing Self-Reported Health Among Rural Low-Income Women Through Health Care and Social Service Utilization: A Structural Equation Model

TIFFANY BICE-WIGINGTON

Stephen F. Austin State University, Nacogdoches, Texas

CATHERINE HUDDLESTON-CASAS

University of Nebraska, Lincoln, Nebraska

Using structural equation modeling, this study examined the mesosystemic processes among rural low-income women, and how these processes subsequently influenced self-reported health. Acknowledging the behavioral processes inherent in utilization of health care and formal social support services, this study moved beyond a behavioral focus by shifting attention to the affective and cognitive processes within the mesosystem. Findings from this study demonstrate that behavioral processes alone did not have a direct significant effect on self-reported health problems over time. However, by shifting attention to the affective and cognitive processes, a missing link between service utilization and future reported health emerged.

Research demonstrates that the incidence, prevalence, morbidity, and mortality rates for disease in rural populations is significantly higher than in the general population, leading to disparities in health among rural residents (Gamm, Hutchison, Dabney, & Dorsey, 2003). Further, among rural populations, the susceptibility to health problems and overall well-being differ by gender and socioeconomic status (Centers for Disease Control and Prevention, 2000). Women living within the context of rural poverty confront multiple interrelated challenges to their health and well-being. Limited health and social services infrastructure, higher rates of poverty, lower rates of employer health insurance coverage, and a systemic lack of health care providers (Merwin, Snyder, & Katz, 2006) all contribute to the health disparities characteristic of the rural low-income population.

Although improvement in health care access is a central goal across rural communities (Gamm et al., 2003), in isolation these efforts are likely to have limited impact on health outcomes. Research suggests that only between 3.5% and 10% of health outcomes are accounted for by the actual delivery of health care (Hartley, 2004; Williams, 1990). Put in other words, a minimum of 90% of health outcomes must be explained by something other than health care delivery. This suggests that bridging the gap to access will only partially affect the health disparities experienced among rural low-income women. Therefore, understanding the contextual influences on health outcomes among rural low-income women is particularly salient for social work practice, as well as program development.

CONCEPTUAL FRAMEWORK

Building upon what is known about health inequalities from a medical model approach, the predominant framework for examining health disparities, this study provides insight into the contextual influences on health outcomes among rural low-income women through an ecological systems perspective (Bronfenbrenner & Morris, 2006). This perspective provides a holistic understanding of health and well-being, as individuals and the environment are viewed as a unitary system within a particular cultural and historical context (Germain & Gitterman, 1996). Exchanges between individuals and the environment are seen as reciprocal, where influence and change is a fluid process occurring across several layers encompassing societal norms, values, institutional structures, interactions between families and systems, and the family system itself (Bengtson, Acock, Allen, Dilworth-Anderson, & Klein, 2005; Bronfenbrenner & Morris, 2006).

In an effort to understand the contextual influences on health outcomes, we focused on two major components of an ecological model: the microsystem and the mesosystem. The *microsystem* refers to the immediate context of an individual, involving person-to-person interactions and relationships where an individual expresses behaviors, intrapersonal characteristics, and participates in bidirectional interactions (Tacon, 2008). From within the microsystem, the individual is conceptualized as the "primary link" that establishes the existence of the mesosystem. The *mesosystem* represents the interrelationships between settings, providing the connection between structures present in one's immediate microsystem (McIntosh, Lyon, Carlson, Everette, & Loera, 2008; Tacon, 2008). Mesosystems permeate everyday processes through the relationships between individuals, families, and community components.

Despite their description as conceptually discrete phenomena, the boundary between the microsystem and mesosystem was theorized, in this study, to be quite permeable. McIntosh et al. (2008) proposed that the mesosystem actually emerges through behavioral, affective, and cognitive processes of individuals. These processes represent transitory mesosystem experiences allowing individuals to recall interactions and apply them in subsequent mesosystem and or microsystem experiences. In essence, the processes blur the boundary between the two ecosystem levels, creating the mental mesosystem, thus influencing the context of the individual. These mesosystemic processes are observable behaviorally as multisetting participation, as well as affectively and cognitively as *intersetting knowledge* (McIntosh et al., 2008).

The purpose of this study was to assess how contextual factors influence self-reported health problems between Time 1 and Time 2 by examining the mediating effects of multisetting participation and intersetting knowledge among rural low-income women. This study examined two hypotheses. First we hypothesized that multisetting participation would mediate the amount of self-reported health problems over time; secondly that intersetting knowledge would further mediate the relationship above and beyond the mediation that occurred through multisetting participation in turn reducing self-reported health problems overtime.

LITERATURE REVIEW

Multisetting participation entails an individual's physical behavior in two or more microsystem settings (McIntosh et al., 2008). For example, multisetting participation might entail an individual engaging in a support group, volunteering at a child's school, and the utilization of local services. The impact of multisetting participation is measured in the frequency of utilization and by the interactions that occur within the setting. Of interest in this study is the utilization of health care and formal social support services among rural low-income women. Research by Cochran, Skillman, Rathge, Moore, Johnston, and Lochner (2002) found that the rural social support programs did not meet the needs of rural families, due to the lack of flexibility of these programs. Further, emerging research confirms and expands upon prior research identifying time limitations, fear of the unknown, low health priority, and lack of companionship or support as reported barriers to seeking preventative health services among rural low-income residents (Murimi & Harpel, 2010). From their findings, Murimi and Harpel (2010) concluded that low-income rural individuals have a health literacy gap interfering with their utilization of services (p. 280). This literacy gap impedes recipients of formal social support services as they experience difficulties completing paperwork and providing supporting documentation (Hasting, Taylor, & Austin, 2005).

Rural residents are characterized as having an underlying culture of independence and self-reliance. These traits foster personal barriers such as feelings of being stigmatized, socially ostracized, and the target of gossip creating a reluctance to seek formal support services as well as health care (Wagenfeld, 2003). These factors contribute to the underutilization of formal social support and health care services until health conditions cause impairment in daily functioning (Bryant & Mah, 1992; Office of Technology Assessment, 1990; Reading et al., 1997; Strickland & Strickland, 1996; Walker, Lucas, & Crespo, 1994). This underutilization among rural populations results in "unrecognized and undiagnosed problems" (Stamm, Lambert, Piland, & Speck, 2007, p. 300), which in turn, further contributes to health disparities among rural individuals.

Less explicit but equally relevant, *intersetting knowledge* refers to an individual's ability to recall and apply information from one setting to another (McIntosh et al., 2008). For example, a participant of the Women, Infant, and Children (WIC) program is provided nutritional education in one setting. The ability of the participant to recall and apply the skills taught through WIC at the grocery store would be an observable application of intersetting knowledge, as the participant applied information across settings. In this study, the intersetting knowledge of interest is the affective process associated with perceived social support and the cognitive process associated with perceived self-sufficiency.

Understanding social networks within rural communities can be "powerful and effective" when paired with formal social support services (Riebschleger, 2007, p. 207). Rural communities have dense social networks, social ties of long duration, and a shared history among residents (Phillips & McLeroy, 2004). Historically, social support has been identified as an important determinant of health risk, whereas a lack of social support increases the susceptibility to health problems. In their pioneering study of social contact and mortality, L. F. Berkman and Syme (1979) found that individuals with low levels of social contact had mortality rates that were two to four and one-half times greater than those with strong social ties. Although L. F. Berkman and Syme were not studying social support per se, their research documents the importance of social relationships to health outcomes. Research suggests that social support provides access to well-being through its ability to provide a protective barrier during stressful situations or life transitions, as well as enhancing one's personal strengths (Caplan, 1974; McCubbin & Boss, 1980).

Emerging research indicates that low-income individuals who report high levels of perceived social support are less likely to utilize formal social support services despite meeting qualification guidelines (De Marco, & De Marco, 2009). In a study of low-income women, Green and Roger (2001) found that women who believed that they had tangible and belonging support, or interpersonal connectedness, reported higher levels of perceived mastery and lower levels of stress. Green and Roger further argued that women who established strong social networks demonstrated greater mastery and control over their lives.

Broadly defined, *self-sufficiency* refers to an individual's ability to make use of acquired knowledge and skills to solve problems and productively move forward. Self-sufficiency is frequently associated with economic stability of an individual and is often a latent goal of government subsidy programs. Yet there is not a clear definition or evaluative tool designed to measure levels of self-sufficiency (Hawkins, 2005). Research asserts that self-sufficiency is more than mere financial security, suggesting that it is a process rather than a goal (Braun, Olsen, & Bauer, 2002; Daugherty & Barber, 2001; Gowdy & Perlmutter, 1993). Gowdy and Perlmutter's (1993) research suggests that self-sufficiency reflects dimensions of autonomy, financial security and responsibility, family and self well-being, and basic assets for living in the community. In their research on the impact of community health programs on low-income mothers, Becker, Kovach, and Gronset (2004) defined *self-sufficiency* as an individual's ability to maintain social, political, economic, and psychological control through their access of information, knowledge, and skills. This control allows individuals to define their own needs, find solutions, and move forward to the next need. However, beyond the research of Becker et al., there is no other research explicitly linking the concept of self-sufficiency to health outcomes.

DATA AND METHOD

The sample of 304 women in this study was drawn from Rural Families Speak (RFS). The central focus of RFS, a longitudinal multistate research project, was to assess the well-being of rural low-income mothers and their families during welfare reform. In RFS three waves of data were collected between 1998 and 2000. The larger RFS data set comprises 465 participants from non-metropolitan counties (populations between 2,500 and 19,000) in 14 states[1] across the United States, as identified through the Butler and Beale (1994) coding scheme. Eligible RFS participants were women age 18, with at least one child age 13 or younger, and a family income below 200% of the poverty threshold. The sample for this study comprises the 315 women who completed Wave 1 and Wave 2 of RFS project. Of those 315 women, this

---

[1]Participating were California, Colorado, Indiana, Kentucky, Louisiana, Maryland, Massachusetts, Michigan, Minnesota, Nebraska, New Hampshire, New York, Oregon, and Wyoming.

study utilized only those with full health data at Time 2, resulting in a sample of 304.

RFS participants were recruited through a self-selection process where informational fliers with eligibility criteria were posted at sites that participants might frequent, including Head Start program sites, Medicaid and WIC offices, and adult education sites. To ensure sensitivity to ethical issues, RFS investigators obtained necessary approvals from the Institutional Review Boards of their respective universities. All RFS participants provided consent to participate in the study and were informed of the purpose of the study, their role and definition of participation, their rights, and confidentiality procedures. Across all data collection sites, interviewers trained in the RFS protocol collected quantitative data using standardized measures, as well as qualitative data in semistructured interviews. This article reports findings using RFS quantitative data.

Measures

This study utilized several components of the RFS interview protocol to test the hypothesized relationship between self-reported health, multisetting participation (behavioral processes), and intersetting knowledge (affective processes and cognitive processes). First, self-reported health outcomes of rural low-income women were operationalized using a 29-item scale at Time 1 and Time 2, in which participants responded on a *yes* or *no* basis if they experienced specific health problems (e.g., high blood pressure, diabetes, cancer, depression, joint pain, fatigue, allergies, frequents colds, and headaches). The count represents the sum total of *yes* responses indicating reported health problems.

Second, multisetting participation or the behavioral processes were reflected through a participant's utilization of formal social support services and health care services. The utilization of formal social support services was operationalized using participants' reported participation in six federally funded assistance programs at Time 1 (e.g., WIC, Free or reduced lunch program, housing assistance, energy assistance, transportation assistance, and Medicaid). The count represents the sum total of *yes* responses indicating participation. In other words, a lower score would indicate that the participant is participating in fewer federally based programs. Participation in formal social support services other than federally funded assisted programs was not collected in the RFS data. Health care utilization was operationalized using a continuous variable where participants provided an estimated number of visits to a health care provider within the last 12 months at the Time 1 interview.

Third, to capture intersetting knowledge or the affective and cognitive processes among this sample, a latent variable was constructed utilizing several components of the RFS interview protocol. The affective processes associated with intersetting knowledge, perceived social support, and perceived self-sufficiency were constructed using the Parenting Ladder. The Parenting Ladder, an instrument developed for utilization in a statewide evaluation of the Healthy Start Program in Oregon (Richards, 1998), has a reported reliability coefficient of $\alpha = .87$, reliability for this sample of $\alpha = .856$. The sample of interest in this study comprises women who had at least one child younger than age 13, thus the Parenting Ladder lends itself to operationalize perceived social support and self-sufficiency as the affective processes of interest.

Perceived social support was affectively operationalized using select items from the Parenting Ladder. The six selected items from the Parenting Ladder assess the degree to which the participant has people on whom to rely for support with a 6-point Likert-type scale that ranges from *low* to *high*. Items include other parents for you to talk to, someone to help you in an emergency, someone to offer helpful advice and moral support, someone to relax with, a professional to talk to, and overall satisfaction with the amount of support.

Perceived self-sufficiency was affectively operationalized using select items from the Parenting Ladder, which captured an individual's perceived confidence in parenting. These items were chosen, as the individuals utilized in this study were all currently parenting at least one child. The seven selected items assess the degree of confidence a participant has in his or her ability as a parent from low to high. Items include knowledge of children's growth and development, confidence to know what is right for child, ability to create safe home for child, success in teaching child to behave, ability to find fun activities of interest to child, amount of stress right now, and ability to cope with stress.

Finally, the cognitive processes associated with intersetting knowledge were captured through an individual's report of perceived social support within the community and perceived self-sufficiency as related to the ability to accomplish tasks critical in everyday living. Perceived social support was cognitively operationalized using the community resource component of the Even Start Life Skills and Community Resource Assessment (Richards, 1998). Through a series of 20 *yes* or *no* questions, the community resource component assesses the degree in which participants are aware of available health and social services in their community at Time 1. The total count represents the sum total of *yes* responses indicating knowledge of where to get help within the community, with a reliability coefficient of $\alpha = .888$. Perceived self-sufficiency is cognitively operationalized utilizing the life skills component of the Even Start Life Skills and Community Resource Assessment. Participants responded on a *yes* or *no* basis to questions related to the ability to accomplish tasks critical in everyday living (e.g., obtaining a driver's license, car insurance, car registration, health insurance, checking account, local library card, the ability to write personal checks, manage bills, make family budgets, stretch groceries at the end of the month, applying for credit cards, preparing meals, getting telephone service, working with land-lord, talking to children's teachers, applying for a job, joining local clubs, and creating a personal support system). The count represents the sum total of *yes* responses indicating a participant's perceived level of life skills, with a reliability coefficient of $\alpha = .778$. In other words, as the sum total increases a participant's perception of ability to accomplish critical tasks increases.

Analysis

The purpose of this analysis was to develop a model to determine if multi-setting participation and intersetting knowledge influenced self-reported health among rural low-income women over time. We hypothesized that, first, multisetting participation would mediate the amount of self-reported health problems over time; secondly, that intersetting knowledge would further mediate the relationship above and beyond the mediation that occurred through multisetting participation, in turn reducing self-reported health problems over time. We tested two variables from the RFS data set and developed a latent construct.

Analysis occurred in two steps. First, the relationships between the vari-ables were assessed using bivariate correlations in SPSS (16). Bivariate corre-lations, standard deviations, and means for each of the observed variables are presented in Table 1. Statistically significant correlations are presented at the $p \leq .05$ and $p \leq .01$ levels. Next, separate structural equation models (SEMs) were developed to test each hypothesis using Mplus (Muthen & Muthen, 2009).

Upon the assumption that the variables of interest would affect reported health problems over time, as outlined in the previously stated hypotheses, all models are presented with fully standardized (STDYX) coefficients. Maximum likelihood (ML) was utilized to account for missing data, as ML uti-lizes available data from variables with values to obtain likelihood values of missing data points.

To assess the quality and statistical significance of both models, several fit indices were utilized. Chi-squared (χ^2) was used to test the hypotheses, in that the relationships proposed in both models provided an explanation of the relationship that exist in the data. A nonsignificant chi-squared value indi-cates a good fit, whereas a significant value would indicate that the given model's covariance structure is significantly different for the observed covari-ance matrix (Kline, 2005). Taking into consideration that the chi-squared stat-istic often lacks power when used with a small sample (as in this study), leading to the inability to discriminate between good fitting models and poor fitting models, additional indices were utilized to assess model fit (Kenny & McCoach, 2003). The Comparative Fit Index (CFI) and Tucker Lewis Index

TABLE 1 Standard Deviations, Means, and Intercorrelations Between Study Variables

	Reported health problems at time 1	Utilization of formal social support	Reported visits to health care provider	Knowledge of community resources	Parental confidence	Perceived social support	Life skills	Reported health problems at time 2
Reported health problems at Time 1	—							
Utilization of formal social support	.150**	—						
Reported visits to health care provider	.239**	—	—					
Knowledge of community resources	—	.260**	—	—				
Parental confidence	-.143**	—	—	.149*	—			
Perceived social support	-.220**	—	—	.290**	.424**	—		
Life skills	—	—	—	.575**	.238**	.370**	—	
Reported health problems at Time 2	.792**	—	.237**	—	—	-.120*	—	—
M	4.22	3.46	9.22	16.58	30.82	26.59	14.44	3.69
SD	3.51	1.55	13.54	4.79	4.92	7.54	3.32	3.29
N	287	275	282	234	279	278	217	304

*p significant at .05 level (2-tailed). **p significant at .01 level.

(TLI) were utilized as incremental fit measures. Both indices are similar in nature as each compares the fit of the model to a null model or independence model, respectively. Further, both indices perform well among small samples. In both cases the indices vary from 0 to 1, where indices greater than .90 indicate an acceptable fit for the estimated model (Kline, 2005). Finally, the root mean square error of approximation (RMSEA), which is the measure of incongruence per degree of freedom, was utilized to measure absolute fit (Kline, 2005). An RMSEA less than or equal to .05 indicates close approximate fit, values between .05 and .08 suggest reasonable error of approximation, and values greater than .10 suggest poor fit (Browne & Cudeck, 1993).

RESULTS

Sample Characteristics

Because RFS eligibility criteria specified that participants had to be females, age 18 older, living in families with incomes below 200% of the federal poverty line, and have at least one child age 13 or younger, the sample was relatively homogenous with little variability in demographic variables. Preliminary analysis revealed that among a highly homogenous sample of rural low-income women, there was not enough variability among the demographic variables to statistically influence the hypothesized relationships.

All participants were women, and on average were age 29.5 (range 18–58) at Time 1. A large portion of the participants identified themselves at White (68.1%), followed by Hispanic (18.4%), and African American (6.9%); the sample is representative of the total RFS sample. Participants' educational levels ranged from less than an eighth-grade education to a graduate degree, with 17.8% having some high school education or less, 30.1% of the participants holding either a high school diploma or a General Equivalency Diploma, and 40.8% having either vocational training or attended some college without degree attainment. Further, a large portion of the participants reported either being married (42.8%) or living with a partner (16.1%). The majority of participants reported having 2.26 children residing in their home at the Time 1 interview, and, on average, participants were age 20.9 when they first became a parent. Almost one half of the participants were employed (45.4%) either part- or full-time, with more than one half (64.7%) of the participants reporting having some form of health insurance.

Multisetting Participation

The first model assumes that multisetting participation at Time 1 will mediate the relationship between reported health problems at Time 1 and reported health problems at Time 2. The mediating relationship and results are presented in Model 1, with fully standardized (STDYX) coefficients (see Figure 1). The model perfectly reproduced the covariance structure of the data, as indicated by the fit indices ($\chi^2 = .0558$, $df = 1$, p Value $= .4552$, CFI $= 1.0$, TLI $= 1.012$, RMSEA $= .000$), however the results do not fully support the hypothesized relationship, in that multisetting participation (reported visits to a health care provider and utilization of formal social support services) is not significantly associated with reported health problems at Time 2.

A standard deviation increase in reported health problems at Time 1 is associated with an *increase* in multisetting participation (reported visits to a health care provider, $SD = .238$, $p \geq .001$, and utilization of formal social support services, $SD = .143$, p $> .05$). In other words, an increase in reported health problems at Time 1 among rural low-income women was associated with an increase in multisetting participation; yet multisetting participation was not directly associated with reported health problems at Time 2.

Although the findings did not support the hypothesized relationship between reported health problems at Time 1, multisetting participation, and reported health problems at Time 2, results indicate that mesosystemic processes, specifically behavioral processes, are influenced by an increase in reported health problems.

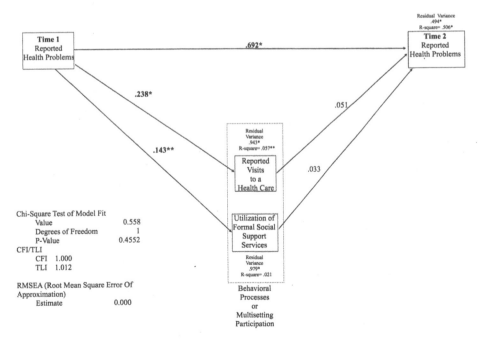

FIGURE 1 Model 1: Multisetting participation. *Note.* Bolded paths are significant. *Significant at .001 level. **Significant at .05 level (2-tailed).

Intersetting Knowledge

The second model extends the prior assumptions, in that multisetting participation influences affective and cognitive processes, processes inherently seen in intersetting knowledge. Thus, Model 2 estimates that intersetting knowledge in Time 1 will amplify the mediating effect of multisetting participation such that, as multisetting participation increases so does intersetting knowledge, and in turn decreases reported health problems at Time 2 (see Figure 2). The results from Model 2 extend the previous findings and are presented with fully standardized (STDYX) coefficients. The model yields reasonable fit indices ($\chi^2 = 35.223$, $df = 17$, p Value $= .0058$, CFI $= .957$, TLI $= 9.28$, RMSEA $= .059$).

The model partially supports the hypothesized relationship, in that a standard deviation increase in the utilization of formal social support services was associated with a $SD = .219$ ($p \geq .05$) increase in intersetting knowledge, when controlling for reported visits to a health care provider. However, when controlling for utilization of formal social support services, reported visits to a health care provider were not significantly associated with intersetting knowledge. Results also indicated that a standard deviation increase in intersetting

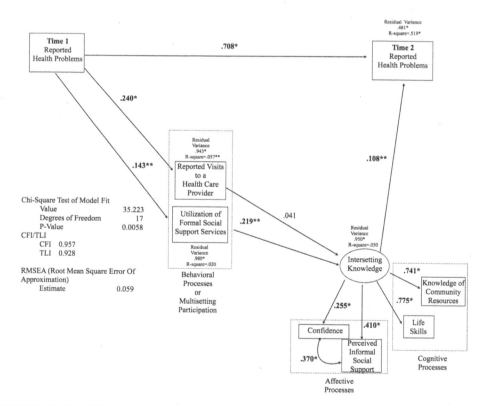

FIGURE 2 Model 2: Intersetting knowledge. *Note.* Bolded paths are significant. *Significant at .001 level. **Significant at .05 level (2-tailed).

knowledge was associated with a $SD = .108$ ($p \geq .05$) increase in reported health problems at Time 2, which did not support the hypothesized relationship.

Although the hypothesized relationship is not supported, it is important to point out the slight decrease in reported health problems over time, t (286) = 3.515, $p < .001$. The first model revealed that multisetting participation was not directly associated with reported health at Time 2. However, the hypothesized relationship between reported health at Time 2 and multisetting participation is established with the addition of intersetting knowledge, as seen in Model 2. This relationship suggests that the behavioral, affective, and cognitive processes of rural low-income women were potentially influenced by reported health problems at Time 1, and moderately influenced reported health problems at Time 2.

DISCUSSION

Findings suggest that the mesosystem is interactional, as behavioral, affective, and cognitive processes directly influence each other. Results of this study support the argument that access to health care and formal social support programs alone does not improve the reported health of rural low-income women. Neither reported utilization of health care nor utilization of formal social support services were found to have a direct significant effect on reported health problems over time. In fact, despite the fact that the rural low-income women from this study utilized slightly more formal social support programs than urban populations (three programs vs. two programs) (De Marco & De Marco, 2009), their higher rate of utilization did not significantly affect future reported health problems. The findings from this study are consistent with prior research suggesting that only between 3.5% to 10% of health outcomes are accounted for by the actual delivery of health care (Hartley, 2004; Williams, 1990).

By moving beyond a behavioral focus on service utilization and shifting attention to the affective and cognitive processes that make up intersetting knowledge, a missing link between service utilization and future reported health emerges. In particular, findings from this study demonstrate that an increase in intersetting knowledge is significantly linked to the utilization of formal social support services, but not to health care visits. Further, increases in intersetting knowledge subsequently increase reported health problems over time. This relationship and the preceding findings suggest two competing interpretations of how the interactional nature of the mesosystem influences health and well-being among rural low-income women.

Intersetting Knowledge Increases Self-Awareness

One interpretation of the findings showing that increases in intersetting knowledge are predictive of increases in reported health problems is that women who possess more intersetting knowledge may also be more self-aware. Perhaps higher utilization of formal social support services enhances intersetting knowledge both affectively, as evidenced by increases in perceptions of social support and reported self-sufficiency, as well as cognitively, as evidenced by increases in life skills and knowledge of community resources. Enhanced intersetting knowledge potentially affords women the ability to make use of acquired knowledge and resources and, in turn, allows them to define their own needs, become self-aware, and be able to better identify health-related concerns.

The conceptualization of intersetting knowledge in both the educational (McIntosh et al., 2008) and medical fields (Campbell & McDaniel, 2000) suggests that intersetting knowledge reinforces mesosystem experiences by linking behavioral, affective, and cognitive processes to unlinked microsystems. This study suggests that the utilization of formal social support programs provided the opportunity for rural low-income women to link mesosystem experiences through intersetting knowledge, thus allowing for affective and cognitive processes to be applied within unlinked microsystems. The use of prior experiences, or intersetting knowledge, affords participants the perception of higher levels of social support and self-sufficiency. Unfortunately, this interpretation fails to explain the lack of significance between utilization of health care and intersetting knowledge.

Rural Independence and Fear of Social Stigma

As previous research has established, rural individuals are often reluctant to access social support and health care services due to personal barriers, a culture of self-reliance, and lack of autonomy (Wagenfeld, 2003). Of the rural low-income women who sought and engaged in more formal social support services and reported an increase in perceived social support and self-sufficiency, it is conceivable that they did not further apply the acquired knowledge and resources in an effort to lessen the perceived stigma associated with their initial utilization of formal social support and health care services. Failure to apply their intersetting knowledge may have contributed to worsening reports of health problems at Time 2.

Previous research on rural culture would lend one to believe rural independence and fear of social stigma prevents multisetting participation, which in turn interrupts the interactional nature of the mesosystemic processes that transfer knowledge to one setting to another among rural low-income women. Although perceived and tangible social support has been linked to higher levels of perceived mastery (Green & Roger, 2001), well-being (Cochran, 2002), and physical and mental health (Seiling, 2006) among rural residents, emerging research suggests that presumed social support associated with individuals living in rural communities might actually hinder access to necessary supportive programs when rural individuals are most vulnerable

(Kelly, Shedlosky-Shoemaker, Porter, DeSimone, & Andrykowski, 2001). When rural low-income women do not feel comfortable making use of support services, other areas in their lives may suffer as a result.

Implications

Results of this study reveal interesting implications for social work practice and education. First, findings suggest that attempts to lessen or alleviate disparities in health and well-being among rural low-income women should embrace an ecological systems approach. This approach would allow social service programs to make use of the behavioral processes involved in seeking, making use of, and conforming to program requirements or recommendations, as well as move service structure toward an integrated holistic approach focused on the interplay between the behavioral, affective, and cognitive processes within the mesosystem to promote health and well-being.

Findings further suggest that a move toward an integrated holistic approach would entail that cultural competency be redefined to embrace an understanding of rural diversity, in that differences are apparent within and between rural low-income women (Riebschleger, 2007).

Rural service providers must not only address the individual needs of their clients but also recognize the rural community context in which clients live and function. For example, a myopic focus on improving access to health care and formal social support services for clients does not automatically translate to improved health within a rural community context. Despite changes in accessibility, rural low-income women continue to confront barriers associated with the stigma of service utilization, as well as low-income status. An understanding of rural culture and the interactional nature of the mesosystem may entail a paradigm shift, moving programs away from linear focused modalities. Recognizing that within the rural context, approaches centered on addressing individual internal and interpersonal processes potentially contribute to the restrictive nature of social service programs and furthers exacerbates the stigma attached with service utilization (Locke & Winship, 2005), subsequently contributing to the differences in health among rural low-income women.

Limitations

As with most research, this study was not without limitations. The sample, although unique in that participants were drawn from a variety of rural communities, was not nationally representative. Participants in this sample were recruited utilizing a self-selection process through local food stamp program sites, Medicaid offices, WIC offices, and adult education sites, which skew findings toward those more likely to participate in formal social support services. Participants were provided incentives to participate in the study. The combined sampling technique, study criteria, and incentive-based participation led to a highly homogenous sample, thus decreasing the variability in factors associated with health risk among rural low-income women. It is also important to note that intersetting knowledge, or the affective and cognitive processes, were assessed utilizing an interview style approach. This approach potentially constrained the responses provided for all of the study measures, thus reflecting either higher or lower levels of reported health problems, multisetting participation, and intersetting knowledge. Finally, and maybe the most critical limitation, health among rural low-income women was operationalized using participants' self-reported health problems, thus lacking the reliability of a standardized measure. However, research demonstrates that over time self-evaluation of one's own health status is considered one of the best indicators of mortality and morbidity (Idler & Kasl, 1991).

CONCLUSION

In summary, this study suggests that within the rural context we must embrace the complexities of rural diversity, as well as recognize the affective and cognitive processes alongside behavioral processes occurring within the mesosystem. With this recognition, we may begin to understand and alleviate the contextual factors associated with rural disparities in health and well-being, among rural low-income women.

REFERENCES

Becker, J., Kovach, A. C., & Gronset, D. L. (2004). Individual empowerment: How community health workers operationalize self-determinantion, self-sufficiency, and descision-making abilities of low-income mothers. *Journal of Community Psychology, 32*(3), 327–342.

Bengtson, V. L., Acock, A. C., Allen, K. R., Dilworth-Anderson, P., & Klein, D. M. (Eds.). (2005). *Sourcebook of family theory and research*. Thousand Oaks, CA: Sage.

Berkman, L. F., & Syme, S. L. (1979). Social networks, host resistance, and mortality: A nine-year follow-up study of Alameda County residents. *Amercian Journal of Epidemiology, 109*, 186–204.

Braun, B., Olson, P. D., & Bauer, J. W. (2002). Welfare to wellbeing transition. *Social Indicators Research, 60*, 147–154.

Bronfenbrenner, U., & Morris, S. (2006). The bioecological model of human development. In W. Damon & R. M. Lerner (Eds.), *Handbook of child psychology: Theoretical models of human development* (Vol. 1, 6th ed., pp. 793–823). New York, NY: Wiley.

Browne, M. W., & Cudeck, R. (1993). Alternative ways of assessing model fit. In K. A. Bollen & J. S. Long (Eds.), *Testing structural equation models* (pp. 136–162). Newbury Park, CA: Sage.

Bryant, H., & Mah, Z. (1992). Breast cancer screening attitudes and behaviors of rural and urban women. *Preventive Medicine, 21*(4), 405–418.

Butler, M., & Beale, C. (1994). *Rural–urban continuum codes of metro and non-metro counties, 1993* (Agriculture and Rural Economy Division, Report No. ERES 9425). Washington, DC: Agriculture and Rural Economy Division, Economic Research Service, U.S. Department of Agriculture.

Campbell, T. L., & McDaniel, S. H. (2000). Consumers and collaborative family healthcare. *Families, Systems, and Health, 18*(2), 133–135.

Caplan, G. (1974). *Support systems and community mental health.* New York, NY: Human Science Press.

Centers for Disease Control and Prevention. (2000). *Measuring healthy days: Population assessment of health-related quality of life.* Atlanta, GA: Author. Retrieved from http://www.cdc.gov/hrqol/pdfs/mhd.pdf

Cochran, C. (2002). A rural road: Exploring opportunities, networks, services, and supports that affect rural families. *Child Welfare, 81,* 837–848.

Cochran, C., Skillman, G., Rathge, R., Moore, K., Johnston, J., & Lochner, A. (2002). A rural road: Exploring opportunities, networks, services, and supports that affect rural families. *Child Welfare, 81*(5), 837–848.

Daugherty, R. H., & Barber, G. M. (2001). Self-sufficiency, ecology of work, and welfare reform. *Social Service Review, 75*(4), 662–675.

De Marco, M., & De Marco, A. C. (2009). Welcome to the neighborhood: Does where you live affect the use of nutrition, health, and welfare programs? *Journal of Sociology and Social Welfare, 36*(1), 141–166.

Gamm, L. D., Hutchinson, L. L., Dabney, B. J., & Dorsey, A. M. (Eds.). (2003). *Rural healthy people 2010: A comparison document to healthy people 2010* (Vol. 1). College Station, TX: Southwest Rural Health Research Center, School of Rural Public Health, Texas A&M University Health System Health Science Center.

Germain, B., & Gitterman, A. (1996). *The life model of social work practice: Advances in theory and practice* (2nd ed.). New York, NY: Columbia University Press.

Gowdy, E. A., & Perlmutter, S. (1993). Economic self-sufficiency: It's not just money. *Affiliate, 8*(4), 368–387.

Green, L., & Roger, A. (2001). Determinants of social support among low-income mothers: A longitudinal analysis. *American Journal of Community Psychology, 29*(3), 419–442.

Hartley, D. (2004). Rural health disparities, population health, and rural culture. *American Journal of Public Health, 94,* 1675–1678.

Hastings, J., Taylor, S., & Austin, M. J. (2005). The status of low-income families in the post-welfare reform environment: Mapping the relationships between poverty and family. *Journal of Health and Social Policy, 21*(1), 33–63.

Hawkins, R. (2005). From self-sufficiency to personal and family sustainability: A new paradigm for social policy. *Journal of Sociology & Social Welfare, 32*(4), 77–92.

Idler, E. L., & Kasl, S. (1991). Health perceptions and survival: Do global evaluations of health status really predict mortality? *Journal of Gerontology, 46*(Suppl. 2), S55–S65.

Kelly, K. M., Shedlosky-Shoemaker, R., Porter, K., DeSimone, P., & Andrykowski, M. (2001). Cancer recurrence worry, risk perception, and informational-coping styles among Appalachian cancer survivors. *Journal of Psychosocial Oncology, 29,* 1–18.

Kenny, D. A., & McCoach, D. B. (2003). Effect of the number of variables on measure of fit in structural equation modeling. *Structural Equation Modeling, 10*(3), 333–351.

Kline, R. B. (2005). *Principles and practice of structural equation modeling.* New York, NY: Guilford Press.

Locke, B. L., & Winship, J. (2005). Social work in rural America: Lessons from the past and trend for the future. In N. Lohmann & R. A. Lohmann (Eds.), *Rural social work practice* (pp. 3–24). New York, NY: Columbia University Press.

McCubbin, H. I., & Boss, P. G. (1980). Family stress and coping: Targets for theory, research, counseling, and education. *Family Relations, 29*(4), 429–430.

McIntosh, J. M., Lyon, A. R., Carlson, G. A., Everette, C., & Loera, S. (2008). Measuring the mesosystem: A survey and critique of approaches to cross setting measurement for ecological research and models of collaborative care. *Families, Systems, and Health, 26*(1), 86–104.

Merwin, E., Snyder, A., & Katz, E. (2006). Differential access to quality healthcare: Professional and policy challenges. *Family and Community Health. Rural Health, 29*(3), 186–194.

Murimi, W., & Harpel, T. (2010). Practicing preventive health: The underlying culture among low-income rural population. *Journal of Rural Health, 26,* 273–282.

Muthen, L. K., & Muthen, B. O. (2009). *Mplus user's guide.* (5th ed.). Los Angeles, CA: Muthen and Muthen.

Office of Technology Assessment, U. S. Congress. (1990). *Health care in rural America* (OTA-H-434). Washington, DC: U.S. Government Printing Office. Retrieved from http://www.fas.org/ota/reports/9022.pdf

Phillips, C. D., & McLeroy, K. R. (2004). Health in rural America: Remembering the importance of place. *American Journal of Public Health, 94*(10), 1661–1663.

Reading, D., Lappe, K., Krueger, M., Kolehouse, B., Stencil, D., & Leer, R. (1997). A cancer screening and prevention in rural Wisconsin: The greater Marshfield experience. *Wisconsin Medical Journal, 96,* 32–37.

Richards, N. (1998). *One step at a time: A report on the outcomes of Oregon's 1996/1997 Even Start Programs.* Corvallis: College of Home Economics and Education, Oregon State University.

Riebschleger, J. (2007). Social workers' suggestions for effective rural practice. *Families in Society: The Journal of Contemporary Social Services, 88*(2), 203–213.

Seiling, B. (2006). Changes in the lives of rural low-income mothers: Do resources play a role in stress? *Journal of Human Behavior in the Social Environment, 13,* 19–42.

SPSS Inc. (2007). SPSS for Windows (Version 16.0) [computer software]. Chicago, IL: Author.

Stamm, B. H., Lambert, D., Piland, N. F., & Speck, N. C. (2007). A rural perspective on health care for the whole person. *Professional Psychology: Research and Practice, 38*(3), 298–304.

Strickland, W., & Strickland, .D. (1996). A barrier to preventive health services for minority households in the rural south. *Journal of Rural Health, 12*(3), 206–217.

Tacon, A. (2008). Approaches to chronic disease and chronic care: From oxymoron to modern zeitgeist. *Disease Management and Health Outcomes, 16*(5), 285–288.

Wagenfeld, M. O. (2003). A snapshot of rural and frontier America. In B. H. Stamm (Ed.), *Rural behavioral health care: An interdisciplinary guide* (pp. 33–40). Washington, DC: American Psychological Association.

Walker, R., Lucas, W., & Crespo, R. (1994). The West Virginia rural cancer prevention project. *Cancer Practice, 2,* 421–426.

Williams, D. R. (1990). Socioeconomic differentials in health: A review and redirection. *Social Psychology Quarterly, 53*(2), 81–99.

Family Caregivers for Seniors in Rural Areas

DEBORAH J. MONAHAN

School of Social Work, Syracuse University, Syracuse, New York

In this article, the demographic characteristics of family caregivers for seniors in rural communities are assessed to examine whether their circumstances could facilitate or impede their well-being. Services available in rural communities for family members providing ongoing care to frail seniors is examined, particularly those that provide health and social services. How families access these services and whether there are specific barriers in service provision are analyzed based on current social work practice and the research literature. Trends for future services are identified as well as whether these trends support new roles for social workers in rural settings.

Caregiving has become a normative phase of the family life cycle in the United States; caregivers report ups and downs in the course of their experience. Research suggests a growth industry in examining the condition of caregivers: their stressors, motivations, consequences, and impacts on family members and the recipient(s) of care. Nevertheless, when resources are scarce and families need to make choices about care, their resiliency may be tipped to a point of needing additional services to restore balance in family functioning. This is particularly evident in family caregiving in rural areas, where services are scattered over larger distances and transportation costs and time can reduce service use. Family caregivers for seniors in rural communities have needs that might lead social work professionals to modify their assessment and intervention decisions in the process of working collaboratively with families and the rural communities in which they live.

In this article, rural family caregivers' demographic characteristics are assessed to examine whether their circumstances could facilitate or impede their well-being. Typical services that are available in rural communities for family members providing ongoing care to frail seniors with an emphasis on health and social services is examined. How families access these services and whether there are specific barriers in service provision is also analyzed, based on current social work practice and the research literature. Trends for future services are identified, as well as whether these trends support new roles for social workers in rural settings.

DEMOGRAPHICS

Care Recipients

Approximately 20% of older persons (age 65+) live in nonmetropolitan communities; older persons living in rural areas and small towns have higher-than-average poverty rates (Administration on Aging, 2011). The National Rural Health Care Association (2002) report from their summit on rural health compared rural and urban elderly and found that rural elderly report worse health, are generally older, have more functional limitations, are more likely to live alone at age 75 and older, are more likely to be "poor" or "near poor," and are at greater risk for long-term care. Growing diversity in rural America and in rural elderly presents an increasing challenge to health, service and aging networks, disputing the "hale and hardy" myth of rural elderly (Buckwalter & Davis, 2011; Krout, 1994). According to Johnson (2005, p. 272), at least two thirds of the nonmetropolitan elderly poor are women. Johnson suggested that outmigration of young people from rural communities results in a concentration of elderly in rural communities. Healey (2004, p. 272) suggested that the cumulative disparities in health status and functional autonomy related to poverty and ethnicity may be particularly stark in rural areas. However, though the health status of elderly rural residents is more complex to summarize, the overall impression is that, after controlling for age, gender, income, living arrangement, and education, the differences may disappear (Johnson, 2005; Redford & Sevens, 1994).

Rural Caregivers

Caregivers often experience strains when their own needs exceed their resources. Spouse caregivers are particularly vulnerable. Overall, rural caregivers are older and in poorer health than their urban counterparts, leading to an increased need for services to bolster their caregiving roles (Buckwalter & Davis, 2011). The Easter Seals Disability Services and the National Alliance for Caregiving Survey (2006, p. 5) of rural caregivers found that 64% are married; 86% are White, 7% Hispanic, 6% Black, and 1% Asian; 25% live in the same household as their care recipient; 41% have children or grand-children; 60% live within a 1-hour drive to provide care; they spend 21 hours per week caregiving, but 19% spend more than 40 hours providing care; and 14% of rural caregivers are Veterans (see Table 1). They reported that the majority (45%) had been providing care for 1 to 9 years, whereas 14% provided care for 10 years or longer. The caregivers' educational backgrounds were varied: 27% have college degrees, 29% completed some

TABLE 1 Profile of Rural Caregivers

Demographic characteristic	%
Marital status	
Married	64
Living with a partner	11
Widowed	6
Divorced or separated	14
Never married	11
Race/ethnicity	
White	86
Black	6
Hispanic	7
Asian	1
Lives with care recipient	25
Distance from care recipient	
Within 1-hour drive	60
One to 2 hours	4
More than 2 hours	11
Caregiving, children or grandchildren	41
Veteran of U.S. military	
Caregiver	14
Care recipient	20
Years providing care	
Fewer than 6 months	23
6 months to 1 year	18
1–9 years	45
10 years or more	14
Education	
Did not complete high school	8
High school or General Education Diploma	36
Some college or technical school	29
College degree	27
Income (in dollars)	
Under 15,000	11
15,000–29,000	17
30,000–49,000	34
50,000–74,000	18
75,000–99,000	8
More than 100,000	11

Note. Adapted from Easter Seals Disability Services and National Alliance for Caregiving (2006).

college or technical school, 36% completed high school, and 8% did not complete high school. Although 11% reported annual income under $15,000, 34% had income in the range of $30,000 to $49,000, and 18% had incomes of $50,000 to $74,000. Although the literature on coping and burden is quite extensive, the focus for this article is on the outcomes for rural caregivers, even though many of the issues may be similar for families providing care to older adults in metropolitan community settings throughout the United States.

Coping and Burden

How caregivers cope with the responsibilities of providing care to an older family member has received considerable attention in the social work and social gerontology research literature (Pearlin, Mullan, Semple, & Skaff, 1990). More recently scholars have focused on the specific outcomes for rural caregivers (Sun, Kosberg, Kaufman, & Leeper, 2010, p. 562) and found that avoidance coping interacted with health to influence caregiver burden. These authors concluded that caregiver interventions could be tailored to rural caregivers' specific coping styles. In a meta-analysis of 78 studies of caregiver interventions, such as psychoeducational, support groups, respite, or psychotherapy, Sorensen, Pinquart, Habil, and Duberstein (2002) reported that the interventions were successful in increasing subjective well-being and alleviating burden/stress and depression.

Greater levels of caregiver burden are associated with a stronger impact of caregiving on caregiver's perceived health (National Alliance of Caregiving and AARP, 2005). Montgomery and Kwak (2008) developed an easy-to-use 32-item questionnaire (TCARE) that assessed three domains of caregiver burden: relationships, infringement on other aspects of life (work, privacy, family), and stress (generalized anxiety). In another study, the Maine Primary Partners in Caregiving (MPPC) project found that caregiving can be isolating and that social workers can encourage family caregivers to develop and sustain their interpersonal networks (Butler, Turner, Kaye, Ruffin, & Downey, 2005). They noted that the social work "strengths-based perspective" can help to identify care tasks and provide social support for rural caregivers.

Relationships in family caregiving are dynamic, and though researchers have studied the "uplifts" or positive aspects of caregiving, the hassles have also been studied extensively (Jensen, Ferrari, & Cavanaugh, 2004; Pinquart & Sorensen, 2003). Early family relationship histories often set the stage for later relationships and may affect the likelihood of the family system to provide emotional support to elderly parents (Whitbeck, Hoyt, & Tyler, 2001, p. 226). The theme of family responsibility has also been examined within the context of caregiver values and norms (Scharlach et al., 2006).

Although this literature is not as well developed for rural caregivers, understanding the complexities of family relationships are an important context in discussing coping and burden.

Family care is provided to spouses, parents, older children with or without disabilities, and other relatives who need social and health services to maintain their independence in the community. When individuals become frail or unable to maintain their independent status, they often call upon relatives to assist them in their daily lives. This support often includes physical and emotional support. These relationships can be positive, and "uplifts" result from these transactions or they can be negative and in severe cases lead to elder abuse or neglect. Emotional abuse has been found to be more prevalent with older women in rural communities than other forms of domestic mistreatment (Dimah & Dimah, 2003, p. 91). Attention to various coping strategies should be investigated further to understand family dynamics in elder caregiving.

Religion as a coping strategy was reported in a study of dementia caregivers in rural Alabama, with White caregivers likely to engage in private religious activities and African American caregivers more likely to engage in organized religious activities (Kosberg, Kaufman, Burgio, Leeper, & Sun, 2007, p. 17). In a related study of coping strategies, the authors reported that "use of religion" was the most frequently used coping mechanism with a score of 15.2 out of a possible 16-point scale, and the authors concluded that "almost all of the rural caregivers used religious coping" (Sun et al., 2010, p. 555). Three indicators of religiosity were found to be inversely correlated with burden in rural caregivers; those who scored lower on caregiver burden were more likely to use religious coping and to be involved in organizational and intrinsic religiosity (Sun et al., 2010, p. 297). Their finding that African American caregivers reported lower levels of caregiver burden than did White caregivers led them to conclude that religiosity serves as a protective function and highlights the roles that different dimensions of religiosity play in the lives of rural dementia caregivers. The authors also suggested that religious activities may provide additional social support and decrease their social isolation (Sun et al., 2010).

Gammon (2000) also suggested that rural churches can be sources of respite care, transportation, and socialization. These are important issues for social workers to assess in determining whether religious affiliation might be identified as a potential resource for programs and services that are relevant to the needs of families. Although social workers may not be as comfortable asking questions about religious affiliation as they are asking questions about "other types" of community affiliation, religious affiliation may be helpful in expanding services for rural caregivers. The types of services that are most typically used by rural caregivers are presented next.

Service Needs

Demographic characteristics such as age, race, and rates of poverty are often associated with service need and use. Although ethnic diversity may be smaller in rural areas, ethnic composition and diversity may have significant implications for social dynamics, local needs, and services (Pugh & Cheers, 2010, p. 9). According to Wilken and Stanback (2011) rural caregivers have the typical needs of other caregivers such as help with physical caregiving; dealing with medical professionals; medication and nutrition concerns; financial, legal, and insurance issues; affordable housing; and managing family relationships; however, there are generally fewer formal services, and they rely more heavily on informal supports. Services used by rural caregivers include counseling, home health services, case management, needs assessment, and transportation (Healy, 2004; Wilken & Stanback, 2011). Support groups have also become a popular service for caregivers to learn more about the roles and tasks associated with family care (Monahan, 2011, p. 32).

Another important framework for understanding services for rural elderly examines six program attributes including their availability, accessibility, adequacy, affordability, appropriateness, and acceptability (Krout, 1994). Johnson (2005, p. 278) stated that the absence and inadequacy of transportation options in rural areas remains one of the most intransigent problems of health and social service delivery for the elderly. Similarly, shortages of health care personnel and the limited number of rural hospitals and medical clinics reduce access to rural elderly and their families. Those available are often strained to provide services that may not be fully funded (Johnson, 2005; Redford, 1998). Social work practice with rural families is often characterized by challenges in responding to client needs such as poverty and isolation, thus requiring an innovative approach to defining and responding to service needs (Buckwalter & Davis, 2003–2004) particularly when they are not aware that they are eligible to receive services or they are reluctant to ask (Butler et al., 2005).

Special needs populations have also been studied in rural communities, particularly those with disease-specific characteristics, such as dementia, that may require more medical attention and carefully designed interventions. Edelman and Kyrouac (2006, p. 230) reported that caregivers for family members with memory loss wanted more information from health providers about the disease trajectory and care implications and that the care recipients had more interest in attending support groups than did the caregivers. Another "special" population of rural caregivers is men; there are not many studies of their circumstances. However, Sanders (2007) reported that male rural caregivers were not as comfortable asking for help and that they needed more instrumental than emotional care. Caregivers for elderly adults with developmental disabilities also face challenges in finding resources for their family members and often feel isolated (Gammon, 2000). Service planning for these special populations is fundamental to well-being of rural family caregivers.

PLANNING EFFECTIVE PROGRAMS TO ASSIST RURAL CAREGIVERS

By understanding the context of rural caregiving, social work practitioners can begin to consider the structural domain of practice and how it affects caregiver well-being. As discussed previously, the needs and characteristics of the caregiving dyad are essential to assess as the foundation for understanding this dynamic care relationship. Families provide care, but the nature and amount of care may vary due to difficulties in their personal lives. Reliance on social and health services in the community to supplement their care is essential. Buckwalter and Davis (2011) identified five critical components necessary to develop effective programs for rural caregivers: relevance, unity, responsiveness, access, and local leadership. By using this acronym (RURAL) to access program effectiveness, social workers can more readily evaluate the needs of caregivers through a more in-depth assessment. Buckwalter and Davis also examine whether programs should be aimed at prevention, client diversity, reducing service barriers, facilitating communication for long-distance caregivers, and the type of personnel needed. Wilken and Stanback (2011) also emphasized that a thorough needs assessment can be done in collaboration with key informants such as public health nurses, health care providers, representatives of the local senior citizens center and staff at Area Agencies on Aging (AAA). Efforts to understand how to improve and evaluate services in rural communities will enable social workers to improve the quality of their referrals and reduce service barriers. Continued funding of federal initiatives for family caregivers is critical to easing the burden of service demands that can be expected to increase as baby boomers begin to use services (Monahan, 2011, p. 40). Difficulties in accessing services and service barriers for rural caregivers are summarized next.

ACCESS AND BARRIERS FOR RURAL CAREGIVERS

Rural caregivers are often at long distances from their relatives/parents and face particular difficulties in rearranging their home and work schedules to provide care. In a MetLife (2004) survey of long-distance caregivers, they reported missing an average of 20 hours of work per month and spending $392 per month on travel expenses to provide care for their parent. The importance of outreach to African American rural caregivers was examined in the Families Who Care project that developed a comprehensive culturally sensitive training packet to increase participation with minority caregivers and their families (Coogle, 2002). They acknowledge that outreach efforts in rural communities may be challenging due to the lack of trained professionals, distance, and service scarcity as well as the isolation of rural families. Another effort to reduce barriers was the Tele-Help Line designed to provide telephone supportive service and outreach using a manualized 8-week intervention to reduce caregiver burden (Dollinger, Chwalisz, & O'Neil Zerth, 2006). The program also incorporated cultural sensitivity in its recruitment and training to respond more appropriately to the needs of ethnic/minority older adults. In a study using focus groups, participants identified several critical service barriers for caregivers that included reliance on informal support networks rather than formal services, lack of knowledge about available service providers, and unavailability of culturally appropriate services (Scharlach et al., 2006, p. 143).

Transportation limitations in rural communities are a major barrier to service access. Approximately 40% of households in rural communities have no public transportation available to them and 25% report insufficient transportation (Park et al., 2010). Access to affordable transportation affects quality of life and the caregivers' ability to access services. The health profile of rural caregivers showed a high prevalence of obesity that raised concerns about the stresses of caregiving and researchers recommended providing counseling to help caregivers understand the importance of self-care (Castro et al., 2007). Access to respite services may also be limited in rural communities; however, rural caregivers who used respite services had the potential to incorporate more service use in their care (Montoro-Rodriguez, Kosloski, & Montgomery, 2003). Rural caregivers also confront structural barriers that limit access to services such as the lack of qualified professionals, a more narrow range, and a more limited supply of services for in-home and community-based services (Li, 2006). Researchers will continue to examine these issues to understand how to increase service access and reduce barriers to vital services for rural caregivers and their families.

TRENDS IN RURAL CAREGIVING AND ROLES FOR SOCIAL WORKERS

As interventions are developed in the future, trends will follow the current trajectory of an increasing population of elderly living in rural communities and their families living at greater distances. Successful interventions for rural caregivers will incorporate a theoretical foundation, an appropriate balance of treatment amount and intensity, and a clearer relationship between treatment and outcomes (Talley, Chwalisz, & Buckwalter, 2011, p. 236). Intervention trends have implications for targeting social work roles from micro- to mezzo- to macro-practice. Social work practice in rural America is an exciting arena from the standpoint of using advanced technology in the 21st century to link people and programs in ways that have been difficult due to the geography of nonurban areas. Social workers can connect with family members and caregivers to coordinate services at a distance using the newest technology to reduce some of the barriers. From teleconferencing to Skype-interviews, listservs, chat rooms, bulletin boards, e-mail, online support groups, and counseling sessions, social workers have tools that can be used selectively to enhance communication (Monahan, 2011; Wasko, 2011).

The use of online and other technologies can facilitate communication with families but also raise ethical issues for social work practice in rural areas. Social workers need to consider how to apply the Code of Ethics to work with clients living in small communities and how confidentiality is protected. (Table 2 summarizes the knowledge and skills for social work practice with rural caregivers.) Maintaining client autonomy while at the same time considering how to promote beneficence, the duty to take action to benefit others, is often challenging (Healey, 2004). Trying to balance a clients' right to self-determination and risk assessment, particularly for frail older adults living alone, requires careful assessment, planning, and communication with clients and family members involved in their care. The assessment of client safety requires a comprehensive understanding of their housing circumstances, its adequacy, and how the client manages decisions about meal preparation, cooking, cleaning, and other situations affecting daily life that require self-sufficiency.

Knowledge about clients may also be learned informally due to the dual relationships that social workers may have in small communities where face-to-face interactions could occur with clients in stores and restaurants, and other places of business or recreation. Dual relationships are sometimes unavoidable and occur when the social worker "assumes a second role with the client" becoming social worker and neighbor or business associate; therefore, these relationships need to be managed to set appropriate

TABLE 2 Knowledge and Skills for Social Work Practice With Rural Caregivers

Knowledge	Skills
Caregiver stress/burden/depression tests	Clinical depression assessment of stress/ burden/depression
Community norms	Community needs assessments
Ethnicity and cultural diversity	Culturally relevant interventions
Family dynamics	Family assessment, therapy
Technology for practice	Online support groups
Dual relationships	Assessing Code of Ethics implications
Normal aging	Tailoring treatment plan to age group
Theories of practice	Implementing treatment with fidelity
Community resources	Case management
Caregiver religious affiliation	Networking for extension of services
Family service utilization/ needs/barriers	Cultural competence and norms in service utilization
Elder abuse/neglect	Interventions targeted at abuse prevention

Note. Adapted from Lohmann and Lohmann (2005) and Talley, Chwalisz, and Buckwalter (2011).

boundaries (Galbreath, 2005, pp. 106–107). An approach to evaluating dual relationships developed by Barnett and Yutrzenka (2002) addresses the importance of documentation, remaining cognizant of confidentiality, and making referrals to other professionals. According to Healy (2004, p. 280) a concern for rural practitioners is the possibility that dual/multiple relationships may influence decisions that disempower older adults living in rural communities. Helping to support the older client maintain their dignity while balancing the risks associated with living alone may challenge relationships with family caregivers whose assessment of risk may differ from the social worker's.

CONCLUSION

Overall, social work practice with rural family caregivers requires thoughtful assessment and monitoring by skilled social work professionals. A strong theoretical grounding in a family-centered, strengths-based, and generalist practice perspective (Lohmann & Lohmann, 2005) is desirable and yields the most effective results. Many structural components of work in rural communities can be considered in the assessments but may not be amenable to alteration. Finding creative ways to navigate the community requires sensitivity to cultural diversity and community norms of practice. Ethical issues are important to examine in planning prior to intervening due to the nature of face-to-face interactions that may occur in small towns and rural areas where personal encounters coincide with professional interactions. Attention to reasonable boundary issues may avert dual relationships during the course of working with rural caregivers and their families. Likewise, when using online support groups, special attention is necessary to avoid violation of client confidentiality.

Evidenced-based interventions to further assist rural caregivers will be developed in the coming years, and the field is open for the creative use of technology. This will be an exciting time for social work practitioners to use their skills in generalist practice to respond to the direct service needs of clients as well as to the planning, implementation, and evaluation of these interventions. The development of an evidenced-based approach to practice with rural caregivers is on the horizon. As researchers continue to study family caregiving there are ongoing methodological issues to consider in the analysis intervention efficacy to effectively meet the needs of rural caregivers. Future social work interventions could include more longitudinal studies, more rigorous outreach efforts to include larger and more diverse sample sizes, and the use of more in-depth qualitative interviews to supplement survey data (Goins, Spencer, & Byrd, 2011). Further research is also needed to increase understanding of the specific needs of ethnic/minority caregivers in rural communities and how to reduce their burden.

REFERENCES

Administration on Aging. (2011). *A profile of older Americans, 2011: Geographic distribution.* Retrieved from http://www.aoa.gov/AoARoot/Aging_Statistics/Profile/2011/8.aspx

Barnett, J., & Yutrzenka, B. (2002). Nonsexual dual relationships in professional practice, with special attention to rural and military communities. In A. A. Lazarus & O. Zur (Eds.), *Dual relationships and psychotherapy* (pp. 273–286). New York, NY: Springer.

Buckwalter, K. C., & Davis, L. L. (2003–2004). *Elder caregiving in rural communities.* Center on Aging. Retrieved from http://www.centeronaging.uiowa.edu/archive/pubs/Elder%20Caregiving%20in%20Rural%20Communities.htm

Buckwalter, K. C., & Davis, L. L. (2011). Elder caregiving in rural communities. In R. C. Talley, K. Chwalisz, & K. C. Buckwalter (Eds.), *Rural caregiving in the United States* (pp. 33–46). New York, NY: Springer.

Butler, S. S., Turner, W., Kaye, L. W., Ruffin, L., & Downer, R. (2005). Depression and caregiver burden among rural caregivers. *Journal of Gerontological Social Work, 46*(1), 47–63.

Castro, C. M., King, A. C., Housemann, R., Bacak, S. J., McMullen, K. M., & Brownson, R. C. (2007). Rural family caregivers and health behaviors: results from an epidemiologic survey. *Journal of Aging and Health, 19*(1), 87–105.

Coogle, C. (2002). The families who care project: Meeting the educational needs of African American and rural family caregivers dealing with dementia. *Educational Gerontology, 28,* 59–71.

Dimah, K. P., & Dimah, A. (2003). Elder abuse and neglect among rural and urban women. *Journal of Elder Abuse and Neglect, 15*(1), 75–93.

Dollinger, S. C., Chwalisz, K., & O'Neil Zerth, E. (2006). Tele-help line for caregivers (TLC): A comprehensive telehealth intervention for rural family caregivers. *Clinical Gerontological, 30*(2), 51–64.

Easter Seals Disability Services and National Alliance for Caregiving. (2006). *Caregiving in rural America.* Retrieved from http://www.easterseals.com/site/DocServer/Caregiving_in_Rural-compressed.pdf?docID=50643.

Edelman, D. K., & Kyrouac, G. A. (2006). Information and service needs of persons with Alzheimer's disease and their family caregivers living in rural communities. *American Journal of Alzheimer's Disease & Other Dementias, 21*(4), 226–233.

Galbreath, W. B. (2005). Dual relationships in rural communities. In N. Lohmann & R. Lohmann (Eds.), *Rural social work practice* (pp. 105–123). New York, NY: Columbia University Press.

Gammon, E. A. (2000). Examining the needs of culturally diverse rural caregivers who have adults with severe developmental disabilities living with them. *Families in Society, 81*(2), 174–185.

Goins, R. T., Spencer, S. M., & Byrd, J. C. (2011). Research on rural caregiving. In R. C. Talley, K. Chwalisz, & K. C. Buckwalter (Eds.) *Rural caregiving in the United States* (pp. 103–130). New York, NY: Springer.

Healey, T. C. (2004). Ethical practice issues in rural perspective. *Journal of Gerontological Social Work, 41*(3/4), 265–286.

Jensen, C. J., Ferrari, M., & Cavanaugh, J. C. (2004). Building on the benefits: Assessing satisfaction and well-being in elder care. *Ageing International, 29*(4), 88–110.

Johnson, C. (2005). Demographic characteristics of the rural elderly. In N. Lohmann & R. Lohmann (Eds.), *Rural social work practice* (pp. 271–290). New York, NY: Columbia University Press.

Kosberg, J. I., Kaufman, A. V., Burgio, L. D., Leeper, J. D., & Sun, F. (2007). Family caregiving to those with dementia in rural Alabama: Racial similarities and differences. *Journal of Aging and Health, 19*(1), 3–21.

Krout, J. (1994). An overview of older rural populations and community-based services. In J. Krout (Ed.), *Providing community-based services to the rural elderly* (pp. 3–18). Thousand Oaks, CA: Sage.

Li, H. (2006). Rural older adults access barriers to in-home and community-based services. *Social Work Research, 30*(2), 109–118.

Lohmann, N., & Lohmann, R. (2005). *Rural social work practice.* New York, NY: Columbia University Press.

MetLife. (2004). *Miles away: The MetLife study of long distance caregiving.* Retrieved from http://www.caregiving.org/data/milesaway.pdf.

Monahan, D. J. (2011). Utilization patterns of caregiver education and support programs. In R. W. Toseland, D. H. Haigler, & D. J. Monahan (Eds.), *Education and support programs for caregivers: Research, practice, policy* (pp. 29–43). New York, NY: Springer.

Montgomery, R., & Kwak, J. (2008). TCARE: Tailored caregiver assessment and referral. *Journal of Social Work Education, 44*(3), 59–64.

Montoro-Rodrigues, J., Koslowki, K., & Montgomery, R. (2003). Evaluating a practice-oriented service model to increase the use of respite services among minorities and rural caregivers. *The Gerontologist, 43*(6), 916–924.

National Alliance for Caregiving and AARP. (2005). *Caregiving in the United States.* Retrieved from http://www.caregiving.org/data/04execsumm.pdf

National Rural Health Care Association. (2002). *Setting the pace for rural elder care: A framework for action.* Alexandria, VA. Retrieved from http://pace.techriver.net/website/download.asp?id=575

Park, N. S., Roff, L. L., Sun, F., Parker, M. W., Klemmack, D. L., Sawyer, P., & Allman, R. M. (2010). Transportation difficulty of black and white rural older adults. *Journal of Applied Gerontology, 29*(1), 70–88.

Pearlin, L. I., Mullan, J. T., Semple, S. J., & Skaff, M. M. (1990). Caregiving and the stress process: An overview of concepts and their measures. *The Gerontologist, 30*, 583–591.

Pinquart, M., & Sorensen, S. (2003). Associations of stressors and uplifts of caregiving with caregiver burden and depressive mood: A meta-analysis. *Journal of Gerontology: Psychological Sciences, 58B*(2), P112–128.

Pugh, R., & Cheers, B. (2009). *Rural social work: An international perspective.* Portland, OR: Policy Press.

Redford, L. (1998). Public policy and the rural elderly. In R. T. Coward & J. Krout (Eds.), *Aging in rural settings: Life circumstances and distinctive features* (pp. 267–286). New York, NY: Springer.

Redford, L., & Sevens, A. (1994). Home health services in rural America. In J. Krout (Ed.), *Providing community-based services to the rural elderly* (pp. 221–242). Thousand Oaks, CA: Sage.

Sanders, S. (2007). Experiences of rural male caregivers of older adults with their informal support networks. *Journal of Gerontological Social Work, 49*(4), 97–115.

Scharlach, A. E., Kellam, R., Ong, N., Baskin, A., Goldstein, C., & Fox, P. J. (2006). Cultural attitudes and caregiver service use: Lessons from focus groups with racially and ethnically diverse family caregivers. *Journal of Gerontological Social Work, 47*(1/2), 133–156.

Sorensen, S., Pinquart, M. Habil, D., & Duberstein, P. (2002). How effective are interventions with caregivers? An updated meta-analysis. *The Gerontologist, 42*(3), 356–372.

Sun, F., Kosberg, J. I., Kaufman, A. V., & Leeper, J. D. (2010). Coping strategies and caregiving outcomes among rural dementia caregivers. *Journal of Gerontological Social Work, 53*(6), 547–567.

Talley, R. C., Chwalisz, K., & Buckwalter, K. C. (2011). Rural caregiving: A quilt of different colors. In R. C. Talley, K. Chwalisz, & K. C. Buckwalter (Eds.), *Rural caregiving in the United States: Research, practice, policy* (pp. 233–267). New York, NY: Springer.

Wasko, N. H. (2011). Wired for the future? The impact of information and telecommunication technology on rural social work. In N. Lohmann & R. A. Lohmann (Eds.), *Rural social work practice* (pp. 41–72). New York, NY: Columbia University Press.

Whitbeck, L. B., Hoyt, D. R., & Tyler, K. A. (2001). Family relationship histories, intergenerational relationship quality, and depressive affect among rural elder people. *Journal of Applied Gerontology, 20*, 214–229.

Wilken, C. S., & Stanback, B. (2011). Strategies to support rural caregivers: Practice, education and training, research, policy, and advocacy. In R. C. Talley, K. Chwalisz, K. C. Buckwalter (Eds.), *Rural caregiving in the United States: Research, practice, policy* (pp. 197–211). New York, NY: Springer.

Barefoot, Country, and Nappy: Life Lessons of a Colored Girl

NORA CHAMBERS CARTER

Winthrop University, Rock Hill, North Carolina

The area of town where we lived was "Black Bottom." The name was given because there were no streetlights in the area. At night, you couldn't see your hand in front of your face. I thought the name came from being a Colored community. We had no idea how poor we were. Though I left our neighborhood long ago, the simple messages are timeless and invaluable. I long for the peace and simplicity of those times. I owe any positive impact made on children in care to the education the Bottom gave her people.

The small town where our neighborhood was located was in Eastern North Carolina. This rural hamlet couldn't boast of a huge population, but my hometown was large enough for me. Everyone in our all Colored neighborhood looked the same, talked the same, acted the same, and believed the same. The "Black Bottom" was a tight knit community and the world as I knew it. The Bottom offered anything that anyone would ever need; most people wouldn't dream of leaving.

BLACK BOTTOM

I grew up in a family of nine children, small when compared to other families in the area. Most families in the Bottom had two parent guardians living in the home. Some children lived with their grandparents when their parents moved to a larger city for a better life. These children usually wore the latest fashions to school due to their parents being exposed to the latest trends. The larger cities offered better jobs and more money. My maternal grandfather, PaPa, spent most of his time in Washington, D.C. and would send money back home to support my grandmother and their three children, including my mother. MaMa, as my grandmother was called, worked taking in washing for other people. As badly as her fingers were curled from arthritis, the additional income was a blessing. Their house was one of the few in the Bottom with a telephone (S. Chambers, personal communication, April 28, 2012).

The Old House

We lived next to our grandmother in a house we referred to as "The Old House." Eleven family members lived in this three-room house. The Old House had a living room, kitchen, and one bedroom. I slept mostly with my parents in the living room on the pull-out sofa. My siblings slept in the bedroom. That room held a double bed and two twin beds. Due to the house not being insulated, the bedroom also had a fireplace that provided heat throughout the winter months. There were times when we would bake sweet potatoes in the ashes. The living room had a wood stove used for heating as well as cooking. The kitchen held a sink, a table, one chair, and a gas stove that was used for heating and cooking. Just outside the backdoor was a pump where we would draw fresh water and a smokehouse for meat. At the end of the property, there was an outhouse.

Although my father worked as a brick mason and on various building projects, our home was dilapidated. When it rained, buckets were placed on the bed to catch the water. Eventually, enough money was saved to purchase a house in the same neighborhood. The day after we moved into our new home, a "condemned" sign was placed on the front of the old house.

Carefree Days

A typical day during the summer months included jumping ditch banks, playing hide and seek in the cornfields, and catching fireflies in mason jars after the sun went down. Other days were spent chasing the guinea fowl, ducks, chickens, rabbits, and goats at my aunt's house next door. We had a garden and were given duties to complete before our parents came home from work.

One of the highlights of summer was when the spray truck came to rid the neighborhood of mosquitoes. Kids would follow the spray truck from neighborhood to neighborhood on their bikes, playing and running through the thick smoke. We found out later that the substance they were spraying was called DDT. Little did we know what we were inhaling or of its possible side effects.

When we were asked to come and rest from our running and playing, we were expected to sit quietly and not offer anything to the adult conversation. It was an unspoken rule that "children were made to be seen, not heard."

The Backyard Bounty

The milkman delivered fresh milk in jars to our doorstep; however, that didn't stop my brother from occasionally milking my aunt's goat. The majority of our food came from our area or nearby farms. This included the meat, as well as the vegetables eaten. My aunt kept animals as pets; however, the chickens were fair game when my father wanted a meal of chicken and dumplings. In addition, most of the families in the community had gardens, especially if your family had a substantial amount of free child labor as we did. The families nearby shared freely of their bounty of vegetables, butter, and milk. Most of the vegetables not sold by farmers were given away. Many of the farmers nearby would leave their fields open to the public after their harvest. Cotton from the fields could be utilized for extra pillow and quilt stuffing, cabbage was used to make chow chow pickle, and fresh corn from the fields nearby helped to make any meal complete.

Our family didn't waste anything: rinds from watermelon were made into pickles and grape hulls were turned into jelly. Had it not been for the creative minds of my parents, we would not have survived. They were able to take basic items and transform them into items that could be used over again.

Mother worked at Flora MacDonald College, an institution for White females, as an assistant in the dining room. This position awarded us additional opportunities for fancier food. When the College hosted a party, we would wait up for her to return home in anticipation of new things she would bring for us to eat. The potential for chicken wings and tea sandwiches were worth the wait. Sunday meals were always special due to Mother having that day off from work. Those meals consisted of what is referred to today as comfort food. Large meals with more expensive food, such as a turkey or ham, were reserved for holidays, such as Easter, Thanksgiving and Christmas. One thing I knew for sure was that we would always have food on the table.

Tonics and Natural Remedies

I went barefoot throughout much of the year and stepped on plenty of rusty nails. All neighborhood children knew how to treat a nail wound with a quick remedy nearby. We would wash the wound with turpentine and cover the area with a piece of salt pork. Rags were wrapped around the foot to keep the meat in place. This treatment prevented soreness from setting in. It seems as if turpentine was given for just about everything. Once home from school, I was given a spoonful of turpentine and sugar. This was supposed to cure whatever was ailing me. It seemed that every child in the neighborhood had worms, most likely due to the poor sanitation conditions. Turpentine, as well as some form of tonic, would help you to pass worms. These remedies were also given to infants.

From spider webs used as a blood clotting mechanism to using leaves as band-aids, there was always something in nature that could be utilized to help cure wounds. These remedies were nothing strange to us or to others within our community. There wasn't much need for a doctor, other than to deliver a baby, and for that, a community midwife lived nearby. For more serious illnesses, I remember overhearing that one of my siblings had gone to the doctor in our town. Unlike one of the restaurants and drugstores downtown, this office didn't only cater to White patients. Everyone sat in the same area as they waited for treatment.

Social Groups and Negative Labels

Blacks were treated as one social group. It was felt that if you did something well, you were a credit to your race. Rev. Dr. Martin Luther King was a leader among Blacks. He was educated and he presented well. Although he was viewed as a peaceful leader, Malcolm X was labeled as violent. He could never rid himself of that negative label in our neighborhood. Often within general conversation, Blacks were questioned by White townspeople as to which of the two leaders, Malcolm or Martin, were preferred. Despite your preference, it was always better to communicate liking Dr. King better than Malcolm X. Within the same conversation, it was nothing for a Black man to be called *boy*, or a woman to be called a *gal*.

Going downtown was still a highlight, and we would look forward to doing so on Saturdays. We would put on our finest clothes, and I would wear shoes. Even then there were stores my Mother refused to enter. She said they belonged to racists or Ku Klux Klan members, and she wouldn't support them with her money. One store owner told my mother that he would eat parched corn for a year to get slavery back. According to my mother, his daughter felt the same way about the desire for slavery to return (S. Chambers, personal communication, April 28, 2012).

It was during one of these trips downtown that I began to experience the ugly truth of the world. I had been allowed to go to the post office by myself. As I was crossing the street, I was called *nigger* by adults who were driving by. There is something about that word that makes your skin crawl; you never know what actions may follow the term. I didn't tell my family about the incident for fear I wouldn't be able to go into town again by myself. That incident has taught me many things, though the incident was long ago. I find that I am cautious in unfamiliar settings. Although I would love to think the world has changed, I still find the world not being kind to children.

Integration and Civil Rights

I was the first in my family to begin my formal education in an integrated school. I hadn't experienced anything different, so the transition into school didn't affect me in any way. Many didn't think integration was a good thing. They worried that integration would never allow a Black valedictorian or salutatorian. Still there was the expectation among many of the people in our community that you didn't cause trouble, that you spoke well and that you walked with your head up high. Mixed-race education was confusing to many of the older students. During the day it was the expectation that you would come together in school as a body of students. The movie theatre downtown had a different set of rules for the evening hours. Blacks were not allowed to sit downstairs and watch the shows (S. Dickerson, personal communication, April 28, 2012).

Integration came at a time when the Civil Rights movement was becoming more violent and forceful. This was a scary time for my family, because my sister had moved to Washington, D.C. prior to the race riots that ensued after Dr. King's assassination. To be in the big city at that time was exciting due to everything going on; however, there was still concern with a small town girl being so far away. Many people in our town had become more transient and were moving to larger cities, especially recent high school graduates. Despite Vietnam War news from my brother-in-law and the many hate crime assassinations, my parents always kept the appearance that none of the many things going on in the world would affect our neighborhood. At the same time, the Black Power movement existed and would have ensured equality, though it would not have been a peaceful process. Not only was James Brown's song, "I'm Black and I'm Proud," political, but it gave the okay to wear your hair without chemicals and to have full lips.

Beauty Symbols

At that time, *dark skinned* and *beautiful* never existed in the same sentence. Media images we saw (long wigs we called falls and light-skinned people) were just the opposite of what was seen in the mirror. The images of beauty on television and in magazines didn't look like me. Symbols of beauty were of super-slim, fair skinned Afro American or White women with blond hair. I began to understand why fairer skinned Afro American people would pass for White. There were different opportunities for them. Our parents taught us that beauty was only skin deep, and my father never missed an opportunity to let us know that he thought we were the most beautiful girls in the world.

In the late 1960s, Diahann Carroll had her own television show. Her popularity began to change the way we viewed ourselves as women. Though she had a lighter complexion, she was the representation of black on television. By this time, my eldest sister also left home for Washington, D.C. and began modeling. She fit the profile of beauty as was displayed by the media. We couldn't wait to get photographs of her, the fashionable apartment she'd rented, and news of the wonderful life she now led.

Not until the 1970s did I began to see beauty represented in darker-skinned people. By that time, we were becoming exposed to magazines such as *Ebony* and *Jet* publications. They displayed minority beauty in ways we would have never dreamed. Naomi Sims was the first African American supermodel. Although she was beautiful, we had a lot of questions as to what it meant to have a dark-skinned person representing beauty. We felt that now we would be taken more seriously or given more opportunity to prove ourselves equal.

TAKING SHAPE

Being the youngest of nine children carried with it a lot of pressure into young adulthood. By the time I began senior high school, I had formulated my own opinion of how I would allow myself to be treated. Many of the teachers, however, had a predetermined view of who I would be, usually based on the sibling they had taught previously. I set about making a conscious determination of who I would be and really liked who I was becoming as a young adult. This stage of life was also met with being bullied and picked on for how I spoke, as well as how I looked. Some students said I spoke "like I was White," and therefore I must have thought that I was White. Others said I was shaped "like a white Girl"—most of us who participated in track and field were more on the lean side. Nevertheless, I couldn't allow any negativism to keep me from the course I had set for myself, to be the best that I could be and to explore other areas.

I entered college with the goal of changing the world. Although I became pregnant in college, I was able to complete my undergraduate degree within 3 years. Prior to attending college, I was denied work because I didn't have a college education. After college, I was told that I was overqualified, though I had no experience. Social work positions in those days were held primarily by White women. They were the ones who would drive the government cars to the houses of families receiving assistance.

My parents didn't qualify for assistance, always making just a few dollars over what was needed to qualify. Giving the conditions in which we lived, my mother was angry that our family didn't qualify for assistance. At the same time, I wondered if my parents would have accepted any assistance from the government or other local programs if it were available.

Financial Support Needs

As a young parent, there wasn't much assistance offered for someone who wanted to work full-time. I felt as if I would have received aid more readily had I not wanted to become employed. Asking for help was embarrassing and degrading. I felt as if the social workers had a personal bias against the needy. Based on my background, I felt that I could have made a difference in the lives of persons applying for assistance. I was in the same boat as many of these people, and I hated being there. Medicaid was beneficial, and I appreciated this aid when my son suddenly came down with an illness that threatened his ability to clot blood. Had it not been for support, I wouldn't have been able to pay for his inpatient stay at Duke University Hospital.

Therapeutic Support Needs

I've often said that Duke represents my greatest hope as well as my greatest loss. The hope being their ability to assist me through my son's illness, the loss represented by another child born 4 years later. Duke physicians were unable to save my youngest son, due to some internal organs not having properly developed while I was pregnant. As with any pregnancy, you enter the hospital with the intention of giving birth to a healthy child and returning home with him. That was not the case, and the experience was extremely traumatic. As a mother, I felt guilty and replayed the pregnancy term over and over in my mind. I wondered what I could have done differently. He was transported to Duke for intensive care, and I was transferred to another floor of the hospital where there were no infants and children.

Grief and loss programs didn't exist in our town. After my son's death, I went through a deep period of depression. Upon a return visit to my doctor, he asked about the support group he thought I was attending. I told him I didn't know of any and hadn't been contacted about becoming involved in any type of therapy. Apparently, this support program was located in one of the larger cities nearby. After realizing that my hair was beginning to fall out, I knew I had to help myself. I had another son, and I needed to start living again. For the most part, no one dared bring up the topic of death, and everyone left me to myself. No one knew how to help me, and so they left me alone. Had it not been for my spirituality, I believe I would have spiraled into clinical depression. At the time of the baby's death, I was working in a day care center in another city and didn't want to return there. I began to look into teaching positions within the school system in our town.

Although I wasn't able to get a full-time job within the school system, I was able to work as a substitute teacher full-time, filling in for teachers during extended illness, office work, and maternity leave. This work cut off additional social program benefits but allowed me an opportunity to teach my son at home and not have an additional day care expense. Unfortunately, I was unable to find employment within the social service agencies in the nearby cities. At the close of the school year, I packed up my belongings and my son and headed to a metropolitan city to find work. It was there that I met my husband. Being married later in life with a blended family is different from the traditional family I grew up in long ago. Although my family tree has changed and the last names are not the same, we aren't much different from one another. My definition of *family* has changed over the years. Family comprises those who sit at a common table, but aren't necessarily connected by blood.

MIDLIFE REVIVAL

I am in the middle of a midlife readjustment. What some would determine a midlife crisis, in terms of my return to school for a master of social work degree, is actually one of the dreams on my to-do list. Baby Boomers are beginning to turn age 65 at a higher rate and will continue to do so until 2030. They may be able to identify better with a peer in supporting them in their senior years. Also, with concerns about the majority of senior citizens not having saved adequately for retirement, having lost their retirement through the economic downturn, and the possible end of Social Security, I'm planning for the next phase of my work life. More importantly for me, I am at a place where I realize my mortality, and I want to give back to the world a legacy of the things I hold dear.

Taking Time for Myself

Earlier in my life, there never seemed to be the right time to return to school. I never took time to do what I wanted to do for me. I was a wonderful cheerleader for others to follow their dreams, but I always found a reason to not encourage myself. In Maya Angelou's book, *Wouldn't Take Nothing for my Journey Now*, she talks about giving herself a day away from the cares of the world. According to her, when she returns, she finds that most of life's questions have been answered. That's how I feel. I didn't put off going back to school, I simply gave myself a day (Angelou, 1993).

The Sandwich Generation

At the time of this writing, my mother is age 88. She is fiercely independent and lives in her home, though with some assistance. She has always inspired us to educate ourselves in every area. Additionally, my mother-in-law has a live-in caregiver, but has been able to remain in her home as well. With six grandchildren, I am a card-carrying member of the sandwich generation.

My grandchildren are another reason I felt the need to return to school for a social work degree. I want them to see that you can accomplish anything you set your mind to do. I would like to remove the word *can't* from their vocabulary, with respect to achieving their goals. I also want them to know that it is their duty to care for other people in this world who are less fortunate than they are. Marian Wright Edelman read a poem at a luncheon years ago about a child who had nothing. This "Greenless Child" she spoke of went about life uncelebrated. This was a child no one wanted to take the trouble to help (Edelman, 2008). I don't want my grandchildren to "tolerate" anyone, because that term carries with it such a negative connotation, in my opinion. I want them to respect others and to know that the responsibility of the "Greenless Child" rests on me today, but that duty will soon be passed on to them.

SELF-AWARENESS AND SOCIAL WORK PRACTICE

One of the greatest things that could have happened to me was growing up in a small town in a small community. I was born at the right time on this journey. "Barefoot, Country and Nappy" describes the carefree lifestyle I loved as a child. I am the sum total of my life's experiences. All of the adolescents in the Bottom were the same and, due to the era in which we lived, our parents had the same expectations of everyone. They wanted their children to go further than they had as parents. It wasn't strange for a parent to admonish a neighbor's child. Everyone in the community was expected to watch out for one another's families, and if something went awry, you were usually called on it. There were no strangers or talk of being in someone else's business. This has changed; many of my neighbors, I don't even know. Then, life was carefree; there was an equal balance of shared work and responsibility. Although some adolescent girls did get pregnant, it wasn't strange to see girls of that age playing with dolls. Most of our parents were within the same income level and educational level. We were all given the same message, to listen to and obey our parents and what they said. In a small community where everyone had everything in common, it was easier to hear the same message from house to house. We were taught that we were no better than any other person and at the same time taught that we were just as good as anyone else.

Although times were simple, I can't always refer to them as the good old days. My parents struggled to make ends meet. They were able to, largely due to community support of friends and family. That ongoing help was dependable. I wonder how our life could have been different with external assistance from social programs. I've always wondered if there was a social worker in our town.

A Mother's Prayer

Mother prayed that nothing would happen to her children. She hoped that she would see her children grown and not depending on others to take care of them. She had seen sibling groups separated in the loss of a primary parent. She'd seen the hardships many of the children faced and didn't wish that experience on anyone. It was easy to see the lack, but what we did have was a strong sense of family and neighborhood connectedness. With so many visible deficits, it would have been easy to miss the less tangible things. My family did the best they could with the hand we'd been dealt. We didn't complain. We didn't realize how poor we truly were until we had a comparison. By that time, we had all left the home place.

Looking back, I guess the community itself served as the social institution. Basic needs such as clothing, shelter, and food were met. Childcare was available through a senior citizen or older sibling. There were times when families would take in someone else's child until the family could get themselves together. For each of those things the community offered, there is now an institution that provides the respective service.

If my life serves for nothing other than deep laughs and wonderful experiences, I certainly have had plenty. There have been many ups and downs, but they all have helped to further develop who I am. Needless to say, "I wouldn't take nothing for my journey now." I became interested in the area of child welfare based on the impact of my early childhood.

Based on my humble upbringing, I don't think there is any client's home that I could step into and not feel some familiarity with having been there myself. From watching stars through the ceiling, to now having more house than I will need, I can identify with any dwelling.

Messages From Childhood

One of the things that all my teaching won't erase are the early messages from childhood that are still in my mind. Even today, I struggle with the perception of laziness. Idle hands were the devil's workshop, we were told. We weren't allowed to sleep late, even on Saturdays. When my Mother would allow us to do so, my Dad would argue that she was "training us to be lazy." Laziness produced weaknesses in people. Often during the summer, farmers would employ schoolchildren to help them in the cucumber fields. My siblings would leave early in the morning and return at dusk. I would plead and cry to go with them, but my Mother thought I was too small. We never questioned the authority of our parents so I never went with my siblings to the fields. Everyone in our community had a job, as well as two or three trades. The simplest thing for any parent to do was to provide basic shelter and food for their family.

Joblessness didn't exist in the Bottom because you always had a trade that you could fall back on. Freedom of expression looked a lot like irresponsibility and like a precursor to laziness. Everything was important and needed to be attended to right then; no time to be frivolous. I have had to make a conscious effort to challenge myself when I meet someone who fits this profile. I was taught to be a workaholic—that was due to my parent's upbringing. They felt this teaching would ensure our survival. Others may not have been taught as we were. Their life lessons don't mean they're lazy, just different than me. I have sought out diversity work to become more culturally competent.

Cultural Competency

Being culturally competent is part of a lifelong journey. Once you think you know something, a situation occurs that causes you to think differently. My family composite has changed significantly over the past couple of years. It has grown to include persons of Latino, White, and Asian descent. Years ago, these interracial marriages and biracial children would have caused quite a stir in our home town. Thankfully, mind-sets have changed more to allow this without fear of harm or death. Our dinner table has welcomed many extra seats; the atmosphere is far from boring. This has led me to choose houses of worship that represent an appreciation for all people. I attend a church with refugees from various cultures who have had to flee their respective countries due to persecution. This too has increased my sensitivity with respect to ethnic sensitive practice.

Learning New Things

My experiences have also helped me to realize we are not too different from other people; we just need to take time to understand that. Too often we don't strive to better understand the reasoning behind a practice before jumping to a conclusion. My granddaughter was sick with fever, and the remedy by her grandmother left marks that looked as if she'd been abused. When I was shown the procedure by her maternal grandfather, it opened up a different world of understanding. This medicinal remedy, treated by rubbing limes repeatedly on the skin of the patient, is no different than the spider webs and leaves I used as a child.

I have an opportunity to change the world, through work with clients. Dr. Nancy Boyd-Franklin believes the most important process in working with families is building a therapeutic relationship with the family. Although she addresses this topic in her work with Black families, it's important for all families. This opportunity also allows us to explore ourselves and our values, perceptions, and cultural similarities and differences that have an impact on our personal frame of reference and on our work (Franklin, 1989).

Other than my age, not much has changed with me. I still want to save the world and all its people; however, I am comfortable with doing so through the people with whom I come in contact. I have seen so many miraculous things happen in my life, and I believe they would not have occurred without divine intervention. God exists and has had a hand in my life from my childhood. Recent interventions were needed to help me revive my life, as well as my career. I had almost gotten to the point where I was suffering from compassion fatigue and was becoming robotic in my work. I had almost forgotten why I entered the field of child welfare in the first place. One of the book's I read during this time was by a gentleman from Cameroon, Africa. In his book, *A People after God*, Denis Ekobena believes that the faith of a person brings them to the realm where impossible things become possible. He further believes that natural things are interwoven within the supernatural (Ekobena, 2009).

I owe a debt to the world based on the opportunities, or blessings, I have been afforded. Although there has been trauma, tragedy, and hardships in my life, I have risen above the circumstances to become stronger. Some would call it resiliency, I say it was God.

Prayers of Support

Like my mother, I pray for my family as well as other children I encounter. I have worked with children in care, and when possible, home is the best placement. Support can sometimes make all the difference in the world to a family struggling to make ends meet. This support doesn't necessarily have to come via financial assistance. There are times when human support becomes more valuable than money. Repayment for my many blessings has become my legacy to those for whom I provide care through service work. I have a strong faith that if I share with clients what I have been taught, coupled with the life lessons given to me, that is my legacy, my reasonable service to the world. I pray even more for the field of social work, that those who truly have a need to improve the conditions of the oppressed will become committed practitioners.

REFERENCES

Angelou, M. (1993). A day away. In *Wouldn't take nothing for my journey now* (pp. 137–139). New York, NY: Random House.

Edelman, M. W. (2008). A letter to our leaders about America's sixth child and the cradle to prison pipeline crisis. In *The sea is so wide and my boat is so small: Charting a course for the next generation* (pp. 77–95). New York, NY: Hyperion.

Ekobena, D. (2009). A people of prayer. In *A people after God: A journey of renewed passion for intimacy with God* (p. 71). Concord, NC: World Changers Publishing.

Franklin, N. B. (1989). Therapist's use of self and value conflicts with Black families. In *Black families in therapy: A multisystems approach* (pp. 95–120). New York, NY: Guilford Press.

The Strengths of Rural Social Workers: Perspectives on Managing Dual Relationships in Small Alaskan Communities

HEIDI BROCIOUS, JACQUELINE EISENBERG,
JENNY YORK, HELEN SHEPARD, SHARON CLAYTON,
and BRITTANY VAN SICKLE
Department of Social Work, University of Alaska Fairbanks, Juneau, Alaska

Social workers are advised to avoid dual relationships; however, this recommendation is not realistic for rural social workers. Using qualitative analysis, this study examines the perspectives of 10 rural social workers in Alaska who are long-term members of their community. From the data, four themes emerged: (1) Rural social workers cannot avoid dual relationships, (2) Healthy dual relationships can have benefits for clients, (3) Social work and other professional education helps rural social workers manage complex situations, and (4) Rural social workers use complex critical thinking and have developed advanced skills to negotiate dual relationships.

Rural social workers are faced with ethical challenges related to dual relationships every day. The majority of research regarding dual relationships involves urban social work practice and recommends that social work professionals try to avoid the complexity of dual relationships with clients. The National Association of Social Workers (NASW; 2008) Code of Ethics does not provide detailed guidance on how to manage dual relationships; rather, it suggests avoidance as the ideal method. Johner (2006) concluded that, "Whatever form dual relationships take, it is without question that most dual relationships inherently violate the belief in the worth and dignity of all humans" (p. 4). Dual relationships provide some of the most complicated ethical challenges in social work (Daley & Hickman, 2011). Due to differing ethical interpretations of boundary transgressions in general, and dual relationships in particular, the social worker is at risk of damaging his or her professional reputation. The difficulty of interpreting and applying ethical standards is described by Freud and Krug (2002):

> The call line had two unrelated cases in which a social worker applied to foster a child whom the social worker had clinically evaluated. In one case the social worker was fired "for transgressing clinical boundaries," while the other situation worked out amicably and to everyone's advantage. (p. 478)

The preference placed on avoiding dual relationships is not consistent with the strengths perspective that prevails in the field of social work. Although existing literature often focuses on the negative aspects of dual relationships, little research has been done to identify possible strengths. This study seeks to identify rural social workers' approach to facing challenges, drawing boundaries, and being effective and ethical in a rural community in the context of dual relationships.

The unique geographic characteristics of Alaska provide an ideal environment to study the issues faced by rural social workers. Most rural Alaskan communities are isolated and are only accessible by air, sea, or vast single-road systems. Almost 15% of Alaska's population is Alaska Native or American Indian (U.S. Census Bureau, 2010). Outside of the main urban areas, the percentage of Alaska Natives is much higher, with some of the highest percentages of native populations in the United States (Ogunwole, 2002). Many rural communities consist of a majority of Alaska Natives (State of Alaska Department of Labor and Workforce Development, 2010). Alaska is home to 231 recognized tribes, with most of these tribes representing individual rural communities (Jaeger, 2004). Referrals in most rural Alaskan communities are not an option.

A common experience in rural Alaska is the itinerant social worker. Because of the extremely small size of many communities, social workers often live in larger communities and travel on an itinerant basis to the smaller villages. This has long been a strategy for providing some level of social work or counseling service to rural and remote communities, but it is a problematic model for several reasons. First, itinerant social workers are often present in the community for only short periods of time, as little as one to two days per month. Second, it is common for a community to have a change in social worker as often as once per year (P. Harding, personal communication, April 12, 2012). Additionally, even when social workers live in the community, it is understood by locals that people who come from "outside" are most often transient and do not plan to stay long term (Alaska School Counselor Association, 2007). This prohibits the community from investing in the itinerant social worker, and the social worker from developing the trust of its members. Communities throughout Alaska have become used to a constant shifting of social work personnel as people move into the State for brief periods of time, then move out because of difficulties adjusting to the isolation, weather, or culture. Social workers from "outside" may not experience the complexities that come with multiple relationships, but any relationship that rural Alaskans forms with them is expected to be temporary (Kennedy, 2008).

The participants in this study represent a newer community response, where local paraprofessionals are supported to earn their social work degrees, reducing the need for itinerant workers and instead developing "home grown" social workers: practitioners that come from the community, know the community, and plan to stay long term. Even with a growing rural workforce, most of the participants have limited or no options for referring clients when dual relationships exist. Instead, these participants are forced to make choices and determine boundaries that allow them to serve their clients and maintain ethical standards that can support long-term efficacy in their communities. Through in-depth interviews, this study examines the perspectives and experiences of 10 rural social workers and identifies strengths-based themes to describe how they are successfully negotiating the challenge of dual relationships.

A small number of articles have identified the frequency with which rural social workers face dual relationships. Gregory (2005) contended that "personal and professional role boundaries are a constant reality in the lives of this cohort. Rural practitioners' lives are a continuous negotiation and renegotiation of boundaries, the properties of which change according to the situation" (p. 261) and further, "the boundaries are not only elastic, but fluid and permeable" (p. 269). The existence of boundary issues and dual relationships are a given, but resources for navigating these ethical minefields are at best ambiguous. Freud and Krug (2002) noted that the rules are subject to interpretation and its subsequent application rests on the discretion of individuals. The Code of Ethics can be confusing to social workers who turn to it as a guide. In addressing limitations, Freud and Krug stated "the Code of Ethics often cannot be used as a guide to ethical practice because of the limitations inherent in any rulebook (p. 477). This places the burden of ethical decision making on the practitioner.

The NASW (2008) noted that building on strengths is a central tenet of the profession. This perspective, however, is most often used to look for strengths in clients who might otherwise be viewed as only having deficits. In this study, we apply the strengths perspective to the client and the practitioner, asking the question, "What are the positive outcomes of dual relationships in rural communities?" and "What resources have developed as a result?" By shifting the conversation, we hope to illuminate how dual relationships are successfully negotiated for the benefit of clients and, further, how avoidance of these relationships may not always be necessary or beneficial.

METHOD

The purpose of this research study was to explore the phenomena of ethical challenges unique to social workers who live and work in rural Alaskan communities—specifically, those challenges related to dual relationships. A qualitative phenomenological approach was used for this study with a focus on lived experiences and perspectives (Creswell, 2007). Semistructured interviews were used to gain a deeper understanding of the rural social workers' experiences and perspectives.

Reflexivity is a critical part of managing research bias and establishing trustworthiness in qualitative findings. For this research, the authors discussed their status as insiders, based on the commonalities of a shared profession and a shared state of residence. *Insider research* refers to when researchers are also members of the population they study (Kanuha, 2000): the researcher shares an identity, language, and experiential base with the study partici-pants (Asselin, 2003). The authors' status as insiders may have contributed to a high level of trust and acceptance by the participants toward the research-ers; it also influenced the researchers' view of the data. Awareness and discussion of shared perspectives as insiders was discussed during work and coding sessions.

Member checking involves corroborating the research findings by seek-ing feedback from the research participants (Creswell & Miller, 2000; Padgett, 2008). In this research, member checking was used; participants were informed that they would be given the first draft of the paper and asked for feedback, clarification, and any concerns about confidentiality. Edits to the paper were subsequently made.

Recruitment & Data Analysis

Based on the research design, a purposive sampling method was used to identify social workers in Alaskan communities with a population of 10,000 or fewer. Participants were identified and recruited through two e-mail list servs, as well as through snowball sampling. Informed consent was obtained for all participants. Institutional Review Board (IRB) approval was obtained for this study through the University of Alaska Fairbanks. Each interview was recorded and then transcribed. Once the data was transcribed, all research-ers participated in an initial coding session of the first transcript, where a basic set of codes were developed. Each remaining transcript was then assigned to two researchers to code individually. This coding was later reviewed as a group to check for consistency. Additional codes were added later as needed. From the initial codes, four themes were derived from the data.

Participants

The 10 participants represented nine different small Alaskan communities ranging in size from approximately 100 to just under 10,000 community members. All of the participants were long-term members of their communities before earning their social work degrees. The ethnicities of the participants were Alaska Native, White, and Asian, with the majority of respondents being Alaska Native. Names and other identifying information, including specifics about ethnicity, were altered or excluded to protect participant confidentiality.

FINDINGS

Four themes emerged from the analysis of the interviews: (1) rural realities: Rural social workers cannot avoid dual relationships; (2) Healthy dual relationships can have benefits for clients; (3) Social work and other professional education and training helps rural social workers manage complex situations they will encounter in practice; and (4) Rural social workers use complex critical thinking and have developed advanced skills to negotiate dual relationships.

Theme 1: Rural Realities: Rural Social Workers Cannot Avoid Dual Relationships

All of the study participants indicated that they deal with some form of dual relationship on a daily basis. These dual relationships may take different forms; they may be service relationships where a client is also one's mechanic or grocery store clerk. Relationships may overlap into areas of the social worker's personal life, such as the social worker having his or her own child share an elementary class with a client's child. Social workers also reported frequent overlap in their social lives, such as attending the same small community celebrations, events, or activities as clients. These events are not occasional but occur on a regular basis for the participants in this study. In rural communities, it seems there is no chance to avoid dual relationships when a community has one church, one mechanic, and one school. For social workers who live in the community, it is more common to have a dual relationship with a client than not: "So the short answer is, yes, pretty much if I left my house I would encounter a client, just going to the store, post office, driving down the road, that sort of thing" (Michelle).

Most participants indicated that their clients know where they live, and how to reach them after working hours. Clients may have known the social workers while they were growing up, or be close to extended members of their family. In some instances, the impacts of these dualities were more complex than simply seeing a client in multiple settings and overlapped into more intricate relationships. One participant, a recovering alcoholic, said that she had to stop going to Alcoholics Anonymous (AA) meetings; her presence at AA wasn't supportive to the clients that she was recommending attend nor was it helpful to her:

> I just remember one of the parents of the kids I was working with, she turned and looked at me and she said, "oh, Ms. Kayla, what are you doing here?" and I knew she felt that I was checking up on her, which, because she had told me she had been going to AA meetings. I never even gave it a thought that I might run into her there, you know. And, so I told her that I am a recovering alcoholic. Of course, neither of us felt real free to share, you know, at that meeting. So I decided at that point that that would not be a source of support that I would use in the community. (Kayla)

Another example of this complexity is that in many communities familial relationships are omnipresent. It is common for residents to be related to a significant portion of the local population, especially in tribal communities. Social workers are faced with the prospect of providing services to members of their extended families:

> There are times that it was a distant relative, and it got to the point where we actually attended the tribal court hearing, and I told our attorney that this is a second cousin of mine, and I just want to disclose it so the whole party knows, everybody involved knows this, and so it was disclosed in the tribal court hearing and everybody agreed that they felt that I could be impartial in representing both [parents] as a caseworker. So you know, and then outside of the office, there isn't necessarily a solid relationship, an acknowledgement that you know you are family, if you happen to be at a funeral together. (Naomi)

Theme 2: Healthy Dual Relationships Can Be Beneficial to Clients

Not only are rural social workers unable to avoid dual relationships, but also many felt there were benefits to their clients as a result of the interwoven relationships within their communities. Participants pointed to cultural competence (an understanding of the history and rhythms of the community and deep knowledge of the community's traditions, beliefs, and behaviors) as a possible healthy outcome of dual relationships. They also reported increased trust (clients knowing who they are and where they come from, plus a long-term commitment to the community) as a possible benefit.

CULTURAL COMPETENCE

Cultural knowledge is extremely important to effective practice in rural Alaska, and many communities have historically been disempowered and disaffected by non-native professionals coming into their communities and providing services in culturally insensitive ways (Kennedy, 2008). This need for cultural knowledge was emphasized by most participants:

> Without any kind of cultural competence and having knowledge of the culture that they are going to deal with, I think you are setting them up for failure. (Michelle)
> I do a lot of community work to promote healing through cultural activities and that is the biggest part of my work, because it's like mass healing, rather than one on one work. (Elsie)
> [When new social workers] are in the community now, they moved here for their position, so as they are getting familiar with the community, the way the community functions, I can definitely see where there is a big gap. (Naomi)
> It might not necessarily be each client that you have all this knowledge about, but it helps that you live with the people. You're part of the people. I see that as a benefit. (Anna)

The social workers interviewed for this study were clear that practice in rural Alaska, without a cultural understanding of the specific community, would be ineffective. They were also clear that to acquire this knowledge to the level they have, overlapping relationships with clients will exist. This is a tradeoff, from their perspective, whereas dual relationships are not without risks, the benefits of cultural and community knowledge almost always outweigh these risks.

TRUST

As described earlier, a common experience in rural Alaska is the itinerant social worker or helper. Because of the extremely small size of many communities, social workers often live in larger communities and travel on an itinerant basis to the smaller villages. This prohibits the community from investing in the itinerant social worker, and the social worker from developing the trust of community members:

> The community knows that I keep things confidential and they have to be able to trust you. That's a big area. If people can't trust you, then, you know, you might as well find another job. But, even in a small community like this, I, the first few year in this job, it was like, people were still

not coming in as often as I would like to see. You know, it took time for them to trust me enough to come in, and have sessions. Even as a community member, and even if they knew that I was trustworthy in matters of confidentiality. I saw testing, I guess you would call it, by the community. Before, you know, it's like, now we're seeing, clients coming more frequently, which wasn't true in the beginning. (Anna)

Theme 3: Social Work and Other Professional Education Make Rural Practice Easier to Negotiate

All participants in this study earned their social work degrees using some model of distance education. Many commented on the impact having a class cohort has had on their ability to manage ethical issues. The participants felt that when academic programs invest in strong peer cohorts, rural social workers may increase their use of supervision and experience a concurrent decrease in their sense of professional isolation.

Participants were included in this study if they had lived in their community prior to earning their social work degree, as this would likely provide a different and more complex experience of dual relationships than for social workers who moved to the community for their job. All but one of the participants were already working in the field prior to earning their social work degrees. Of these nine, all indicated marked improvement in the quality of their work as a result of their educational experience. A commonly identified benefit of their formal education was increased knowledge about ethical practice and managing confidentiality:

> I can tell you that I was judgey and that I would know stuff and I wouldn't be mindful in my own head how I used that information with a client. [before my university education] I didn't have the skills to be able to self-reflect or talk to someone, or to have good supervision to know how to deal with that. (Mia)

Participants felt that their formal education either prepared them well for practice or improved their competency if they were already working in the field. Forming peer relationships and learning the value of using professional and peer supervision were also discussed by many participants as an important way in which they found support to practice effectively in rural communities:

> I was able to be a part of a [school] cohort, so that was my support system that I had built across the state, so I have a big wide web of little resources and friends all over the state. And you know with just the touch of a button or little emails to check in with one of them to say "hey, can you just share with me or what is your opinion about this" and so that is how, having those references and having people in my life that are having similar situations, that is what has helped me figure out how to deal with certain things. (Michelle)

According to participants, focus on the practice of ethics in rural communities specifically was helpful in preparing them for work in the field. They reported that ongoing training directed at negotiating confidentiality with clients has helped them manage relationships in a way that protects the clients, while allowing the service provider to continue to practice effectively in a rural community. Offering these educational opportunities has also increased the effective use of supervision and has helped the rural social worker utilize the resources and knowledge of other experienced individuals.

Theme 4: Rural Social Workers Use Complex Critical Thinking and Have Developed Advanced Skills to Negotiate Dual Relationships

Rural practice adds a layer of complexity to social work ethics, and participants in this study appear to have developed advanced critical thinking skills in implementing the NASW Code of Ethics as a result. Rural social workers negotiate the shades of grey on a daily basis and describe their ethical decision-making process in a variety of complex scenarios. Several common experiences in rural communities provided opportunities for participants to demonstrate their advanced critical thinking, including knowing the client's history, wearing different hats (role distinction), dealing with confidentiality, managing gossip, and negotiating gift giving.

KNOWING THE CLIENT'S HISTORY

Important skills that rural social workers acquire are the ability to critically and carefully examine personal bias in relation to the intimate knowledge of the community, and to deal with the personal knowledge about the lives of their clients: "It's kind of like a juror, [I] kind of have to say, can you look at this without any bias, and I think that is something that you have to develop, it comes with maturity of being in the profession that you are in" (Naomi).

Intimate knowledge of the lives and histories of their clients places an additional burden upon the rural social worker. They must carefully consider which information will be utilized, and which information will be disregarded to assess and support clients. Although social workers cannot erase prior knowledge that is attained through familiarity, they must develop skills to manage that information appropriately and not impact clients in negative ways:

> I usually, if it's something really major, I'll bring it up and just ask the person. But there is a lot that is just hearsay and rumor and whatnot, and I don't bother with a lot of that. In assessments and things like that, I just go with what the client tells me. If I know the person really well and I know something different, then I'll bring it up and go from there, but if they absolutely refuse to admit whatever, then that is where it's at. (Elsie)

As noted earlier, many social workers who are long-term residents of their communities are also related to many community members. For social workers in this circumstance, it was important to make the distinction between close family and extended family. Participants were clear that it was not helpful to act as a social worker for close family, but that working with extended family was a different and often unavoidable matter. The degree to which these fine distinctions are made, and the process the social workers used to make these distinctions, is a clear example of the level of critical thinking rural social workers must use when applying ethics and managing personal bias.

> I have many relatives here in the community and when they are too close, I'll ask to have another counselor come in. If I'm too closely related to the family, I will give them to the other counselor because of the conflict of interest. If it was a relative that wasn't that close, I would let them know, let them understand that there is, I am a professional right now, this is not ... the relationship is different kind of relationship, I have to know that I have a different role in our conversation rather than being related. (Lori)

The rural social workers interviewed for this study generally did not have the option to refer clients when cases of personal bias presented themselves. In these instances, the social workers pushed themselves professionally and personally, practicing the skills of self-awareness and self-reflection to manage these relationships with the best interests of the clients in mind.

ROLE DISTINCTION "WEARING DIFFERENT HATS"

Social workers in this study often discussed the concept of "wearing different hats" to describe how they managed their different roles in the community. This metaphor appears to be used to clarify what they and the clients can expect in different situations. Participants talked about taking off one hat and putting on another when they are in the process of switching roles in the community. For example, they described asking themselves, "What hat am I wearing now?" If it is their "social worker hat," one set of interactions and behaviors is appropriate. If it is their "parent hat," another set of behaviors and interactions must occur. Participants found that they need to be exceptionally clear with themselves what hat they are wearing, and that wearing these different hats requires ongoing communication and education of their clients:

> As you probably know, living in a small community you wear different hats and you have different contacts so for different situations or with different people that I kind of turned to for support. (Allison)
> You know, it's not uncommon that we change different hats when we leave this place [the office]. When I leave my work and I see my clients here, we change a different hat and put something else on. (Michelle)

The rural social workers then use the idea of hats to help clients set boundaries outside the office:

> I learned to do that with every client. I'd tell them when they come in, "When I see you out there, I cannot discuss anything to protect your confidentiality." So that was what I had to learn to do from the very beginning, what to tell the client. Because, you know, in a small community, everybody is really close and thinks it's okay to talk about anything. (Betty)

By setting boundaries based on the situation and the best interests of clients, and consistently maintaining those boundaries in public situations, rural social workers demonstrate increased skills in ethics management and display a complex thinking process about how best to negotiate the dual relationships they inevitably encounter. It is this level of expertise they have developed that can be considered for future study in effective management of dual relationships.

CONFIDENTIALITY

Managing concerns and expectations around confidentiality are among the most common ethical situations negotiated by rural social workers. Study participants commonly reported the following situations: protecting their clients confidentiality, demonstrating their high commitment to keeping information to themselves, and protecting clients even when clients do not protect themselves:

> I learned pretty quickly to be very clear about that it was confidential, very clear about confidentiality and then also I started to try to set really good boundaries about, I wouldn't approach them in public unless it was inappropriate not to say hello. And if somebody tried to talk to me outside of the office about things, too, I would try to direct them back to a confidential way, like coming to my office, or calling me on the phone, that type of thing. I tried to still protect our confidentiality even if they weren't protecting their confidentiality. (Allison)
>
> But when you're out in the community and stuff, because of close personal relationships you have with people, you don't feel like they protect their own confidentiality very well. (Elsie)

The rural social workers in this study developed a system for dealing with these encounters that involved discussing what may happen during a public encounter in initial sessions. This was followed by ongoing efforts in public settings to remind clients of their rights to confidentiality and maintaining boundaries to protect the clients' interests even if the client did not.

MANAGING GOSSIP

In small communities, there is little that happens that does not eventually become common knowledge. Professionals who have lived in the community long-term are not immune to learning secondhand information. Additionally, concerned family members may independently seek the social worker out to share information without the client's permission. The end result is that a rural social worker often has extensive information about a client that did not come through the professional–client relationship. Again, this is a dual relationship issue that is rarely faced by the urban social worker and takes critical thinking and thoughtful bias management to negotiate the situation in an ethical way. These rural social workers were intensely focused on the best interests of their clients in every ethical challenge they faced.

Participants in the study reported different ways of managing gossip. Some social workers try to block it from their minds, letting their clients tell their own stories; others find that gossip must not be ignored and must be discussed with the client when it is a serious matter or involves harmful allegations. Many use critical thinking skills to determine which information they will acknowledge and address, whereas other information will not be addressed unless brought up by their client. Mia felt that it was important to listen to some gossip in order to be a first line of defense. She stated:

> So, say we were worried about some, or the gossip around the village was you know so and so was getting drunk or so and so did this and it was someone under 18, so I might say, well, I'm going to do youth activity and I'll make sure to contact that person and really reach out to them to get them there, and then the [Village police officer] might say, well from my angle, this person needs to do community service, but I'll make an effort to make sure they get there … and we all tried to coordinate to form a safety net under that person.

She also felt that it was important to ensure that prior knowledge of a client's history did not color her perception of her client:

> It makes you biased and you have to try not to be biased even if you know, even if you think you know their story, you have to try to kind of, I want to say scrub it out of your mind, because, it is important to meet someone and let them tell their own story and not walk in there with your misconceptions or preconceived notions because everybody sees things differently and experiences something differently. (Mia)

Allen took a common sense approach to the subject of utilizing gossip. He felt that there were times when hearsay needed to be taken seriously, and other times that gossip was simply not beneficial and should be left to the clients to bring up on their own if they wanted to address it. Allen stated,

> If the client is willing to talk about it, or your situation [is] like somebody is being threatened like it's a sexual abuse or a child abuse, then I'll go ahead and address that because somebody's life is being endangered. But if it's a hearsay that I don't think is going to be beneficial, then you know, I let the person I'm working with bring it up.

Michelle looked at hearsay as a potential indicator of trouble that should never be avoided. Her stance was that ignoring gossip in rural towns was potentially detrimental:

> I think that you do more damage if you don't talk about the issues and you don't address it like we should be, as social workers, that is one of our primary responsibilities is to help service everybody. When you intentionally ignore things, like underage drinking or vandalism, and you keep saying "well that's that families' business," you don't pay attention because it doesn't directly involve you, you are just as guilty as the one that is committing the crime. That is how I look at it.

All of the responses demonstrate nuanced critical thinking skills, self-reflection, and common sense in regard to the use of secondary knowledge with their clients. All study participants seemed to consider that there were instances when gossip needed to be ignored, and instances when gossip needed to be addressed and utilized.

GIFTS

Gift giving, bartering, and simple sharing is also a way of life in many rural Alaskan communities. People share food as a matter of course. The proceeds of a bountiful day on the water, for example, can result in gifts of fish to all people in the village. In many communities, to keep the proceeds of a hunting or fishing expedition for yourself is seen as a shameful act (Condon, Collings, & Wenzel, 1995). Many of the social workers that we interviewed were faced at one point or another with a gift from a grateful client. There are settings and times when gifts are accepted to ensure that cultural traditions are acknowledged or respected, that people are not offended or humiliated, or that one does not give the appearance of being standoffish and aloof.

> We don't, in our culture, this is an area where it is so important to know the culture that you're going into, and I know in the code of ethics it says you shouldn't accept gifts from clients and stuff, but in this community, we're a, I guess you would call it collective community, where

people share, especially when it comes to food. And people share what they get from when they go out hunting or stuff, and it would be an insult if, you know, did not receive that. It would cause, I think, more harm than good. Because, see, motive is different, if that makes sense. Because in certain communities it would not be proper to say, you know, when someone brings you some food, it wouldn't be proper to say "no I can't because of the code of ethics." It would just cause more, um, it wouldn't help. (Lori)

Recognizing that acceptance of certain items because of the cultural nuances did not mean that participants accepted all gifts. Instead, they thought deeply about the meaning and intent of the gift, within the culture of the community, and responded in the way that would be most beneficial to the client:

I also kind of like look at what is the item they are giving me. If it is a lot more than what it is, then I will tell them I cannot take it. I can take this much, but ... so it's more like where I think it's not really like kind of like seeming like they have some other underlying reason for doing that. (Allen)

For participants in this study, a culturally sensitive approach to receiving gifts from clients was warranted, rather than a blanket rejection.

SUMMARY AND CONCLUSIONS

As a central tenet of the social work profession, the strengths perspective can be instructive, not just for working with clients, but also in negotiating ethical dilemmas. This article examines how the strengths perspective can be used to discuss ethical challenges faced and managed by rural social work professionals. As noted, four themes were elicited from the data. These themes provide a realistic and positive frame for learning more about how rural social workers use their skills effectively. The previous focus of research on the negative impacts of dual relationships offers little value to the rural social worker: What benefit is there in recommending avoidance when this is impossible? Participants in this study were able to use the benefits that come with being familiar in the community (e.g., increased trust and community and cultural awareness), while carefully balancing the associated risks by keeping their clients' best interests as their central focus. Participants were disciplined in their practice of using supervision. To this end they continued to use the network of support systems they had developed in their professional education. The participants' commitment to applying the intent of the NASW Code of Ethics allowed them to independently evaluate each situation and respond in ways most beneficial to the people they work with.

Future research needs to focus on the nuanced aspects of this issue; specifically, what are the professional decision-making steps to managing a dual relationship specific to a rural setting? Legitimizing this reality in the profession will allow rural social workers more opportunity to share their knowledge and skills as well as to continue to grow in their abilities and get support when needed. The strengths perspective dictates that we look for the positive aspects of complex issues and utilize resources rather than focus on limitations. This approach can be applied to rural social work and can result in stronger and more effective professional practice.

Limitations

There are several limitations to the study that may impede its transferability to other rural social workers. First, as is the case with many in-depth interview based studies, the sample size is small and not necessarily representative of the population. The unique culture and geography of Alaska, different than other rural areas, may also limit the transferability of the study findings. Other limitations worth considering are that, given the inclusion criteria, all participants earned their undergraduate degrees from the same institution and are former students of the lead author. Finally, it can always be challenging to talk with social workers about ethical dilemmas, because of the sensitive nature of the topic. Participants may have been reluctant to discuss cases or circumstances that were exceptionally difficult, or where they may question their past decision making.

REFERENCES

Alaska School Counselor Association. (2007). *Alaska school counseling framework*. Retrieved from http://www.alaskaschoolcounselor.org/page/ak-school-counselor-framework

Asselin, M. E. (2003). Insider research: Issues to consider when doing qualitative research in your own Setting. *Journal for Nurses in Staff Development, 19*(2), 99–103.

Condon, R. G., Collings, P., & Wenzel, G. (1995). The best part of life: Subsistence hunting, ethnicity, and economic adaptation among young adult Inuit males. *Arctic, 48*(1), 31–46.

Creswell, J. (2007). *Qualitative inquiry and research design: Choosing among five approaches*. Thousand Oaks, CA: Sage.

Creswell, J., & Miller, D. (2000). Determining validity in qualitative inquiry. *Theory into Practice, 39*(3), 124–130.

Daley, M., & Hickman, S. (2011). Dual relationships and beyond: understanding and addressing ethical challenges for rural social work. *Journal of Social Work Values and Ethics, 8*(1). Retrieved from http://www.socialworker.com/jswve/spr11/spr11daleyhickman.pdf

Freud, S., & Krug, S. (2002). Beyond the code of ethics, part I: Complexities of ethical decision making in social work practice. *Families in Society, 83*(5), 474–482.

Gregory, R. (2005).Whispers on the wind: The small quiet voice of rural health and welfare practice. *Rural Society, 15,* 267–273.

Jaeger, L. (2004). *A few differences between Alaska and lower 48 tribes.* Tanana Chiefs Conference, Fairbanks, Alaska. Retrieved from http://www.tananachiefs.org/pdf/Differences%20between%20Alaska%20and%20Lower%2048%20Tribes.pdf

Johner, R. (2006). Dual relationship legitimization and client self-determination. *Journal of Social Work Values and Ethics, 3*(1), 1–11.

Kanuha, V. (2000). Being native vs. going native: The challenge of doing research as an insider. *Social Work, 45*(5), 439–447.

Kennedy, T. (2008). *Where the river meets the sky.* Penang, Malaysia: Southbend Press.

National Association of Social Workers. (2008). *National Association of Social Workers celebrates National Professional Social Work Month in March 2008* [Press Release]. Retrieved from http://www.socialworkers.org/pressroom/2008/012908.asp

Ogunwole, S. U. (2002). *The American Indian and Alaska native Population: 2000* (Census 2000 Brief). Retrieved from http://www.census.gov/prod/2002pubs/c2kbr01-15.pdf

Padgett, D. K. (2008). *Qualitative methods in social work research* (2nd ed.). Thousand Oaks, CA: Sage.

State of Alaska Department of Labor and Workforce Development. (2010). *Alaska population overview 2009 estimates.* Retrieved from http://146.63.75.50/research/pop/estimates/pub/popover.pdf

U.S. Census Bureau. (2010). *State and county quickfacts, Alaska.* Retrieved from http://quickfacts.census.gov/qfd/states/02000.html

Giving Voice to Rural and Urban Social Service Providers: Recessionary Effects on the Provision of Services in Hawai'i

REBECCA L. STOTZER and CHRISTOPHER C. C. ROCCHIO

Myron B. Thompson School of Social Work, University of Hawai'i at Mānoa, Honolulu, Hawai'i

Utilizing an Internet-based survey, 98 administrators, managers, and supervisors in social service settings answered quantitative and qualitative questions about recessionary effects on services and strategies employed to cope with budget shortfalls. Respondents reported making reductions in personnel and programs, with private providers suffering more reductions, and rural counties cutting programs and personnel at higher rates than urban counterparts. Respondents also related concerns about program sustainability, caseload sizes, personnel burnout, impacts to quality, and long-term impacts to clients. Providers utilized a variety of strategies in an attempt to preserve services for vulnerable individuals and their families.

Anecdotal reports suggest that social service providers struggle to address the increased needs of vulnerable families affected by the global financial crisis that began in 2008. Few studies have examined the recession's impact on the delivery and quality of social services, as well as outcomes associated with these changes. Moreover, there is a dearth of information comparing the impact of the economic recession on social services in rural areas. The few examples that were found attributed recessionary effects to increased poverty rates, child poverty rates (Economic Research Service, 2009), and higher rates of unemployment (and subsequent lack of insurance) in rural areas (McBride & Kemper, 2009). These studies suggest that rural families and providers face unique challenges.

Social work, to date, has not adequately explored the impact that the economic downturn has had on rural families or rural providers. This lack of attention to rural areas postrecession confirms a common critique of the profession that social work pays insufficient attention to the full range of social problems found in contemporary rural America (Helton, 2010; Mackie & Lips, 2010; Slovak, Sparks, & Hall, 2011). This is also true in social work practice (Riebschleger, 2007); only 3% of licensed social workers, 2% of health social workers, and 2% of mental health social workers practice in rural areas (National Association of Social Workers, Center for Workforce Studies, 2006), even though 19.3% of Americans live in rural areas (U.S. Bureau of the Census, 2012). Not only is there a lack of social workers, but there is also a lack of social service agencies and programs in rural areas. For instance, Belanger and Stone (2008) found that rural areas are statistically different from urban areas in the number of counties without substance abuse treatment for children and teens, residential treatment for children and teens, school social work, and after school programs. Even when services are available, there is higher per capita spending among nonprofit social service programs in urban areas than in rural areas (Hager, Brimer, & Pollack, 2005). These studies suggest discrepancies in social service availability and direct cost expenditures in rural communities even prior to the economic downturn.

This study seeks to uncover the immediate impact that the economic downturn has had on rural and urban communities by examining data gathered from social service providers in the State of Hawai'i at the end of 2009. A survey was sent to social service administrators, managers, and supervisors as a part of a larger advocacy and policy effort to inform ongoing budget cuts being made by the state of Hawai'i. Specifically, this study examines the strategies urban and rural providers employ to survive in the difficult economic situation. This study also highlights opinions about the impact that these changes will have in communities over the long term.

IMPACTS OF THE ECONOMIC DOWNTURN

The National Association of Social Workers (2009) attributed increased rates of domestic violence, suicide, and depression to the recent global recession. Families' experiences of economic pressure and subsequent maladaptive coping behaviors may explain the rise in the use of emergency domestic violence shelters (Lyon, Lane, & Menard, 2009) and increased utilization of acute behavioral health services since 2008 (Reardon, 2009). The economic downturn has also been linked to increased levels of alcohol abuse (Mossakowski, 2008), decreased ability to pay for health services (Barner et al., 2011), and inability of fathers with child support orders to make their payments (Wu, 2011).

In Hawai'i specifically, there were some early signs of the social impacts of the recession. For example, major crime rates increased (Vorsino, 2010a), in 2010 Hawai'i saw the highest rates of poverty since 1997 (Vorsino, 2010b), unemployment increased 3.6% since the start of the recession (Thomas, 2011), and welfare numbers rose for the first time in a decade in 2009 (Vorsino, 2009). Although the overall outlook of Hawai'i's economic future is not as desperate as some other states (McNichol, Oliff, & Johnson, 2012), the impact of the nation's economic hardship will be long lasting due to Hawai'i's dependence on a tourist economy.

Despite some signs of an economy starting to recover, budget shortfalls forced the State to amend appropriations within each department to account for loss in tax revenues. Given that Hawai'i procures a significant portion of its budget to fund contracts with private providers rather than employ a large public workforce, many of these agencies received notice of significant cuts in a very short time frame, with little chance to secure monies from other funding streams.

In response to policy-related decisions about changes to agencies and programs across the state (including the termination of contracts, the large scale Reduction-in-Force [RIF], and mandatory furlough days of public employees) organizations around the state coordinated efforts to counter the budget reductions. To add data to their advocacy efforts, members of the University of Hawai'i Myron B. Thompson School of Social Work designed a statewide survey of social service managers/supervisors/executives to determine the impact of the budget crisis on social services. Given that only one county in Hawai'i is designated as urban by the U.S. Census and all others are designated rural, understanding the impact of the budget crisis on providers statewide is critical for creating meaningful recommendations for local policy advocacy efforts. The purpose of this study is to uncover the impact the budget crisis has made in rural and urban counties' social services and clients in Hawai'i.

METHOD

Materials and Procedure

To address the impact of the budget crisis on rural and urban counties in Hawai'i, a brief, 46-item Internet survey was distributed across the state targeting supervisors, managers, and administrators working in the social service field. This survey had three main sections, including demographics and workforce competency issues. The focus of this study is on the questions related to the impact of the budget crisis that began in the summer of 2008.

The survey utilized a mixed-method design with quantitative and qualitative measures to gain a broad understanding of the issues in the social service community as well as giving the respondents a chance to identify their own concerns through open-ended questions.

Quantitative questions related to the budget crisis focused on the expertise of supervisors, managers, and administrators by focusing on their impressions of the change in their ability to deliver services following the budget crisis. Participants were asked two yes/no questions. First, whether they had been forced to reduce their workforce, either by laying off or eliminating positions and second, whether they had been forced to make changes to programs, including the possibility of discontinuing services due to budget shortfalls. Participants were then asked a series of four matched questions about their ability to perform in the past and in the present. Given that there was no baseline data, this survey relied on retrospective questions to establish "prebudget crisis" judgments. These were Likert-type scale items that asked respondents to rate how much they agree or disagree (1 = *strongly disagree* – 5 = *strongly agree*) with a series of five statements:

1. Prior to the budget crisis/[Currently] we were/[are] able to carry out the goals and objectives of my program.
2. Prior to the budget crisis/[Currently] we were/[are] able to provide the highest quality services.
3. Prior to the budget crisis/[Currently] caseloads were/[are] very manageable.
4. Prior to the budget crisis/[Currently] we had/[have] enough resources to effectively serve clients.

Qualitative questions focused on the changes respondents experienced in their agency as part of the severe round of budget cuts. Specifically, participants were asked:

1. Given the current economic challenges in the state of Hawai'i, have you had to implement any changes to program delivery? If so, what types of changes have you had to implement?
2. Given the changes that social service organizations have undergone in the current economic situation in Hawai'i, what impact (if any) do you think these changes will have on the long-term quality of your program?
3. Is there anything else you would like to tell us about workforce issues or program delivery issues in the state?

Data Collection

The survey was conducted utilizing SurveyShare, online survey software. The survey was made available to participants from October 1, 2009 to November 14, 2009. Only supervisors, managers, and administrators who were currently working were asked to participate via an e-mail invitation. The invitation e-mail was first distributed among social work students, faculty, and staff at the Myron B. Thomson School of Social Work who were asked to forward the e-mails to their known contacts of supervisors, managers, and administrators via a snowball methodology. The invitation e-mail was also sent to all practicum instructors in the practicum office's contact list, and also via the local National Association of Social Workers (NASW)-Hawai'i Chapter. The invitation assured prospective participants that their identities would remain anonymous if they chose to complete the survey. The survey did not include any questions that would compromise their anonymity. Further, prospective participants were informed that the researchers had disabled the Internet protocol (IP) address collection feature that has the possibility of inferring the participant's specific geographic location.

The State of Hawai'i consists of hundreds of islands forming an archipelago stretching more than 1,600 miles (2,600 km) in the Central Pacific and is the furthest island chain from any landmass in the world. Nearly all of the population resides on eight islands that are at the southeastern end of the chain. These eight islands are divided into five counties: Kaua'i County (the islands of Kaua'i & Ni'ihau), Honolulu County (the island of O'ahu), Maui County (the islands of Maui, Lana'i, Kaho'olawe, & most of Moloka'i), Hawai'i County (island of Hawai'i, also known as "Big Island"); and Kalawao County, a former Hansen's disease colony (located on Moloka'i) (Albrecht, 2008). Of these, the majority of the State's population resides in Honolulu County (the island of O'ahu). The other inhabited islands are called "neighbor islands" and comprise communities designated as rural (and in some cases remote) by the U.S. Census (2012), and are all designated as medically underserved (State of Hawai'i Department of Health, 2012). Due to the historic neglect to the concerns of neighbor island residents and social service programs, particular effort was spent on disseminating the survey to prospective participants in Hawai'i County, Maui County, and Kaua'i County. In particular, students enrolled in the distance education option of the MSW program and in an advanced research class distributed the e-mail to practitioners on their islands. As is typical of a snowball sampling method, there was no way to determine response rates because it is unknown how many people actually received the e-mail invitation. According to the State of Hawai'i Department of Labor and Industrial Relations (2009), although there are roughly 10,000 people working in social or community services, there are only about 660 social service managers in the state.

Participants

The survey was completed by 98 people with an average of 19.4 years of experience in the social service field, and 9.9 years of experience as supervisors, managers, or administrators. The majority of respondents held social work degrees (65.3%), many were licensed (46.6%), and the majority held advanced degrees (82.7%). Respondents were a fair representation of the people of Hawai'i, with Whites (38.8%), Asians (20.4%), and Native Hawaiian/Pacific Islanders (17.3%) making up the bulk of respondents.

The majority of agencies that these respondents represented were private agencies (60.8%) and addressed a wide variety of people and social problems throughout the state. The majority were involved in child and family welfare broadly defined (32.7%), followed by mental health and substance abuse services (19.4%), and violence, crime, and incarceration related services (8.2%). There were also respondents from gerontology settings (9.2%), homelessness/housing agencies (3.1%), medical settings (5.1%), and settings where individuals with disabilities were their primary population (6.1%). Fifty-one percent of the respondents were from Honolulu County, 25.5% from Hawai'i County, 10.2% from Kaua`i County, and 13.3% from Maui County.

Data Analysis

Given the brevity of responses in the online survey format, most answers to each question were fewer than 200 words, making the most appropriate analytic strategy a content analysis. Utilizing a method of constant comparison (Dye, Schatz, Rosenberg, & Coleman, 2000; Glaser & Strauss, 1967; Lincoln & Guba, 1985), five students in the MSW program independently read the responses for a single question and developed codes. Then, they compared categories and worked to reach 100% consensus about what constituted a category. The responses and the newly developed codes were then given to five additional MSW students, who implemented the coding scheme to the original responses. Any discrepancies were brought to the original coding students, until all data points were effectively placed within a category, or discarded (e.g., unintelligible responses).

RESULTS

Quantitative Findings

REDUCTIONS IN WORKFORCE

Participants were asked, using a dichotomous yes/no option, whether they had to eliminate positions because of the current budget crisis. Overall, 43.2% of participants reported having eliminated one or more positions in their organization. When comparing reductions, there was a statistically significant difference ($\chi^2 = 4.04$, $p < .044$) between public and private agencies, with 51.7% of respondents from private agencies and 30.5% of respondents from public agencies having reported reducing their workforce. The highest number of eliminated positions were reported in Kaua'i County and

Hawai'i County, both of which are rural counties. Yet, when comparing rural and urban counties on eliminating positions in response to the budget short-fall, there was no statistically significant difference (marginally significant, $\chi^2 = 2.9$, $p < .08$) between rural (52%) and urban (34%) counties.

REDUCTIONS IN PROGRAMS

Participants were asked, using a dichotomous yes/no option, whether they had to cut programs due to the current budget crisis. Overall, 52% of partici-pants reported having to cut entire programs. Forty-two percent of respon-dents from rural counties and 46% of respondents from urban counties reported program cuts. Reductions did not differ between participants from rural or urban counties or public or private agencies. Similarly, there were no statistically significant differences between public and private agencies, with 54.4% of respondents from private agencies and 50.0% of respondents from public agencies reporting having to eliminate programs.

IMPACT TO SERVICES

Participants reported meaningful declines in their ability to meet program goals and objectives, provide high-quality services, ensure manageable case-loads, and have access to adequate resources (see Table 1). In ratings of the past, most respondents selected *agree* or *strongly agree* across all four domains. However, in their ratings of the present situation, participants were more likely to select *neutral* or *disagree*. Scores dropped from 22% to 53%. The largest declines were in caseload manageability and having adequate resources.

Discussion of Quantitative Findings

The recession clearly impacted public and private providers from rural and urban counties. Altogether, more than 50% of participants reported having to

TABLE 1 Changes From Past to Present

	Score past					Score present				
	1	2	3	4	5	1	2	3	4	5
Able to meet goals & objectives	1	5	3	46	36	4	15	6	47	22
Able to provide high quality services	1	6	6	39	39	5	20	16	30	23
Caseloads are manageable	1	13	14	37	26	9	21	17	35	12
Have adequate resources	1	9	8	43	30	8	29	18	24	15

Note. 1 = strongly disagree; 2 = disagree; 3 = neutral; 4 = agree; 5 = strongly agree.

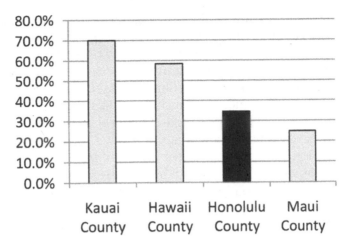

FIGURE 1 Percent of respondents reporting reduction in workforce by county.

cut programs, and 40% reported having to eliminate positions. Despite note-worthy reductions in personnel and programs, the only statistically signifi-cant difference found was between public and private agencies having reported reductions in their workforce. No significant differences were found between urban and rural providers; however, different mechanisms were employed to ensure programs remained viable.

Different strategies were employed among rural counties to cope with the economic downturn (see Figures 1 & 2). For example, Maui County eliminated programs at much greater rates than they terminated positions, suggesting some reorganization of existing workers. In contrast, Kauaʻi County appears to have worked hard to keep program cutting minimal while many jobs were lost. Some of these differences are sure to be related to the

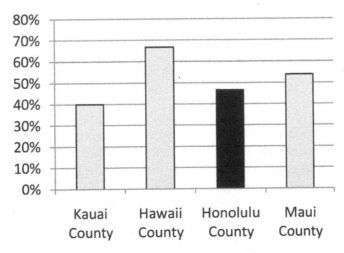

FIGURE 2 Percent of respondents' agencies that had cut program by county.

nature of the funding streams of the organizations in rural counties. In some locations, State funding is one of the few sources of social service revenue, and thus loss of contracts resulted in catastrophic program closures. In other more developed counties, there was a more diverse set of funding opportunities that may have led to more program stability but position cuts instead.

Participants reported meaningful declines in their ability to meet program goals and objectives, provide high-quality services, ensure manageable caseloads, and have access to adequate resources. Results should be interpreted with caution as the retrospective nature of the study may have inadvertently given respondents "rose-colored glasses" about the past while enmeshed in the present budget crisis. Nevertheless, the declines in these scores suggest that agencies are working hard to meet their goals and objectives, but that this may be at the cost of increasing caseloads, decreasing quality, and a loss of adequate resources.

Qualitative Findings

Rich qualitative data offer insights into the types of changes that have occurred. Eighteen percent of respondents indicated not having been financially affected by the economic crisis. Among those who reported no changes in their programs or agencies, 60% of those respondents were located in urban areas, again suggesting a difference in the overall impact of the budget crisis on rural and urban locations, with more rural providers having to assume changes. Among the respondents whose agencies/programs have been affected by the budget crisis, qualitative responses provide a contextualized narrative of the changes and problems the budget crisis has generated. Findings are grouped by the three main qualitative questions: What changes to programs/services occurred because of budget cuts? What was the impact of those changes to program delivery? Are there any other observations about the workforce issues that should be clarified?

Changes to Programs and Services

CHANGING PROGRAM DELIVERY OPTIONS

Forty-eight percent of respondents described having been forced to make a variety of cuts, such as decreasing services, reducing the number of clients served, and reducing salaries. More specifically, 31.7% of respondents reported being forced to make programmatic changes, the most prevalent strategy being a redefinition of those served (e.g., implementing more stringent eligibility standards). One urban provider of a community center reported, "We have had to re-evaluate which clients to serve first. We have also had to cut seven programs and no longer can serve clients in certain areas (geographic and issues)." Another urban provider of an elder-serving program said that their program had to "implement an Urgent waitlist (along with the current Priority client waitlist and non-priority client waitlist)."

REDUCED SALARIES

Respondents also reported having reduced salaries to offset budget shortfalls that otherwise would force staff layoffs or eventual closure of needed social service programs. For example, a rural provider of child and family mental health services said "Supervisor and I took on 3% pay cuts to upper management, 2% pay cuts to middle management (program supervisors), 1% pay cuts to salaried admin, staff mileage reimbursement cut from .42 to .32 per mile."

Changes in job duties/responsibilities and work effort. Twenty-four percent of participants also reported concerns regarding caseload size and activity. Common themes included longer work hours, higher caseloads, redefined positions, and increased need for workers to assume responsibility for shared caseloads. One urban supervisor of a crisis and trauma center wrote,

> Our program currently has to provide more services to more clients than before the budget crisis for the same compensation and with the same number of staffing. Additionally, due to cuts in other programs, this program is seeing more clients than before and the scope of the program is being forced to shift slightly in order to meet the needs of additional clients (often with less services than they had access to before the budget crisis).

One respondent of a child welfare–oriented program in a rural location created a comprehensive list of the changes, "We have had to close cases more quickly to keep case sizes manageable and to focus on high risk cases. Workers have had longer hours." Some reported the use of creative approaches in assuming shared responsibilities and roles in the face of mounting work. For example, one manager reported that they

> collaborated with another program in agency to share a FTE [full time employee] due to budget could only pay for half time position. Then we were able to fill a vacated position (changed position from full time to half time for our program).

Positive outcomes of the budget crisis. Despite these dismal reports, many respondents found some bright spots in the economic circumstances. Some (11.3%) highlighted that more cost effective and innovative practices have been employed given the financial constraints imposed by the budget crisis. One substance abuse director believed that budget shortfalls would "improve the quality [of services]. Those good at their jobs will remain, and those who are not moving clients forward or who are inefficient in their practice will be forced to find other careers."

IMPACT TO PROGRAMS/AGENCIES

Burnout and loss of professionals. Eighteen percent of respondents expressed ongoing concerns about the social service workforce, and the likelihood for burnout and the loss of talented professionals. One program director of a private child abuse prevention organization said that,

> I think increase stress, overall stress and financial stress, will begin taking a toll on everyone. This may increase our referrals and ultimately caseloads. There are a lot of confusing changes that no one seems to know. This lack of knowledge now will cause a snow-ball effect of confusion in the long term.

Declines in quality of services. Some of the more distressing commentary was about the long-term impacts to the social service array. Although many identified how cuts to their own programs and others all constituted a broad weakening of the safety net, 7.6% had serious concerns about declines in quality of services. Thirty-two percent reported significant changes in the quality of their services, such as having longer waitlists, more difficulty getting or referring to other services, shorter lengths of service delivery, and cases being prematurely terminated. For example, one rural provider of geriatric services reported, "Cut back hours has meant less time with clients in need. Increased clients not receiving support and counseling." A rural provider that serves at-risk populations said, "program eligibility ... criteria more restrictive, less families will meet new criteria, which means less families will be served," whereas another rural provider of child and adolescent oriented services added, "referrals are being scrutinized so it harder for kids to be found eligible for our services." When asked about the long-term impact of the current budget crisis on the future quality of their programs, only 13.8% of respondents reported that they did not foresee any more changes that would need to be made, whereas the remaining participants all predicted other critical changes for the future.

Loss of professional development. The impact on social services and the workforce could have long-reaching consequences. Many respondents cited the loss of professional development and no time for supervision, suggesting an additional layer of loss in workforce development. A supervisor from a public child welfare unit said that, "We have had to lay off the less senior workers and are therefore unable to develop the younger workers and build a skilled and seasoned workforce for the future."

Impact on clients and families. Although the survey was specifically asking about workforce and programmatic issues, many respondents (33%)

included information about their perceptions of impacts to clients and at-risk families. One urban respondent of a child and family serving organization said, "The children and families we serve will not receive the utmost care and guidance needed to ensure success in the future." Others identified the ways in which fiscal decisions, such as reducing duplication in services, created additional burdens for at-risk families. For example, an urban child and family serving organization manager said,

> Families have been put on waitlists for services. We lost our in-house MSW that provides in-home therapy and assessment. Now we have to refer out which is difficult for families who don't have transportation or have certain types of insurance.

A mental health administrator had a bleaker outlook on consequences to clients, "Our clients will decompensate and will utilize the hospital more frequently, police involvement will increase, ambulance cost will rise, suicide and homicide rates will increase." Of particular note, 6.4% of respondents (all of whom serve rural areas) specifically described the increase in client deaths as a distinct possible outcome.

A serious concern mentioned in rural and urban settings, though dominated by urban respondents, was the increased number of problems expected due to the increasing stress to families and the decreasing amount of supports in place. Even though this survey was conducted shortly after the state's announcement of their strategies for budget cuts, one urban respondent said,

> The families we work with are facing cuts to many of the services they need to resolve the issues that led to the removal of their children from their home. Mental health, substance abuse, and domestic violence issues are the three most common issues our families face and all of them have experienced a decrease in the amount/quality of services provided.

Many mentioned the increased need for cash assistance as more families fail financially, and increased rates of family violence and other social problems. Three respondents in particular predicted that the loss of most prevention services was going to have a long-term impact on society and social services for years to come, with one saying, "We will be forced to service more families who will be in more serious situations as many prevention services have been cut."

DISCUSSION

Results of the survey suggest that the recession has had a significant affect on social services, as well as those individuals and families being served by social service programs. Overall, urban and rural providers across public and private agencies were forced to reduce their workforce as one of the primary means of coping with reduced budgets. Public and private providers employed different mechanisms to ensure programs remained viable. Supervisors, managers, and administrators across the State also expressed grave concerns about the impact of these changes on their ability to deliver high-quality programs to the State's most needy populations, with particular concern voiced by rural providers for the clients and families in their communities.

Differences emerged in coping strategies between public and private, as well as rural and urban providers. Privately funded social service organizations were more likely than publicly funded agencies to eliminate positions due to budget shortfalls. A number of reasons could account for this difference, including the state modifying or ending contracts with private providers as a budget solution, and the fact that state workers are unionized making the elimination of positions more challenging than eliminating contracts. Private and public agencies in urban and rural settings modified or terminated existing programs to cope with the budget crisis, and private agencies were more likely to have reduced their personnel and their programs. There were no statistically significant differences when examining reductions in workforce and changes in programming among rural and urban settings, possibly due to the small sample size. However, patterns suggest a worrisome level of impact to rural areas. Some providers emphasized securing programming over positions, but no data collected from this survey inquired about the decision-making process.

Qualitative responses detailed a complicated picture of the impact the budget crisis has had on urban and rural agencies. Participants described distressing predictions about the long-term impacts to the array of services across different systems and settings. These predictions of long-term impact were particularly stark among rural providers. Increased caseloads, limited resources (including the availability of qualified professionals to provide supervision), and the unpredictable fiscal environment were mentioned as disconcerting to social workers and human service professionals serving families in rural and urban settings. The evidence of these changes gave providers serious cause for concern, and many discussed the impact to individuals and families in need and predicted long-term consequences to Hawai'i's most vulnerable residents. However, these social work supervisors, managers, and administrators were not giving up; as one urban provider said, "No family should be denied visits due to a lack of revenue." Another provider said simply, "We need to invest now in order to reap the benefits of society in the future." Unfortunately, these providers' predictions about serious impacts to clients were not wrong. For example, under oath, the executive director of an agency providing services in rural and urban settings suggested that more service recipients had died as a direct result from policies implemented by the Department of Health (Capitol TV, 2010).

Study Limitations

The initial intent of this research was to provide information for advocates who were fighting the policy decisions that reduced budgets to social service providers. This led to limitations in the study design such as having questions guided by practicality as opposed to being driven by theory, an incredibly short turn-around time for data collection that led to a smaller sample size than is typically desirable for complex statistical analysis, and no plans for, or implementation of, follow-up surveys to determine the longitudinal impacts of the budget prioritization decisions. However, this survey provides very unique prospective data about the immediate impact of budget cuts in the first year after the onset of the economic recession. The study was also limited by the nature of the retrospective "baseline" pretest used to compare evaluations of the current state of social services in Hawai'i. Although this method has strengths related to response shift bias (Program Design and Evaluation, 2005), this method was chosen due to a lack of baseline rather than the inherent strengths or weaknesses of a retrospective pre-/posttest design. Future studies should consider the bias inherent in answering questions about the past budget situation while in the midst of a budget crisis.

Future Research

Future research should examine how diverse funding sources and a sudden loss of funds affect rural counties in ways that are similar to or different from urban counties. This research should include how those differences among providers in rural and urban counties affect decisions about balancing the reduction of programs and/or personnel. Future research should also examine the impact that the economic recession has had on the delivery and quality of social services, particularly in regard to short-term versus long-term impacts for social service providers and families served by these agencies, as well as outcomes associated with these changes in rural and urban settings.

CONCLUSION

The global financial crisis that began in 2008 will most likely continue to affect individuals, families, and communities in rural and urban settings for many years. This study found that the immediate impact of the budget crisis among social service agencies in Hawai'i resulted in reductions in personnel and programs. Rural communities reported higher rates of being forced to make organizational/program changes, and private agencies were hit harder by budget cuts than public agencies. These agencies and programs demonstrated admirable resilience via a variety of coping mechanisms to deal with the budget shortfall, such as cutting staff, redefining program eligibility, and changing job duties or reducing salaries, not simply cutting programs or personnel. However, these changes also resulted in increased concerns about burnout for social service providers, loss of the ability to mentor or develop professionals, reductions in service quality, and significant affect to clients and at-risk families. The dire nature of the long-term affect of these program changes were particularly evident in the qualitative responses of rural providers, who felt that the inability to adequately serve their social service resource-poor communities would have consequences far into the future.

REFERENCES

Albrecht, D. E. (2008). The State of Hawai'i. In *Population Brief: Trends in the Western U. S.* Retrieved from http://wrdc.usu.edu/files/uploads/Population/Hawai'i_WEB.pdf.

Barner, J., Tetloff, M., Okech, D., Miller, S. E., Clay, K., & Beatty, S. (2011, January). *Tough times: The impact of the recession in Athens, GA.* Paper presented at the meeting of the Society for Social Work and Research Conference, Tampa, FL.

Belanger, K., & Stone, W. (2008). The social service divide: Service availability and accessibility in rural versus urban counties and impact on child welfare outcomes. *Child Welfare, 87,* 101–124.

Capitol, T. V. (2010, March 16). *Hawaii State Senate, committee on health and committee on human services, information briefing on the Adult Mental Health Division.* Honolulu, HI: Olelo Community Media.

Dye, J. F., Schatz, I. M., Rosenberg, B. A., & Coleman, S. T. (2000). Constant comparison method: A kaleidoscope of data. *The Qualitative Report* [On-line serial]. Retrieved from http://www.nova.edu/ssss/QR/QR4-1/dye.html

Economic Research Service. (2009). *Rural America at a glance, 2009 edition* (Economic Information Bulletin Number 59). Retrieved from http://www.ers.usda.gov/Publications/EIB59/

Glaser, B. G., & Strauss, A. (1967). *Discovery of grounded theory: Strategies for qualitative review.* Chicago, IL: Aldine De Gruyter.

Hager, M. A., Brimer, A., & Pollack, T. H. (2005). The distribution of nonprofit social service organizations along the rural-urban continuum. In N. Lohmann and R. Lohmann (Eds.), *Rural social work practice* (pp. 73–85). New York, NY: Columbia University Press.

Helton, L. R. (2010). Faculty perceptions of differences between teaching rural Appalachian and urban social work students. *Contemporary Rural Social Work, 2,* 66–74.

Lincoln, Y. S., & Guba, E. G. (1985). *Naturalistic inquiry.* Newbury Park, CA: Sage.

Lyon, E., Lane, S., & Menard, A. (2009). *Meeting survivors' needs: A multi-state study of domestic violence shelter experiences* (Document No. NCJ 225025).Washington, DC: U.S. Department of Justice, National Institute of Justice.

Mackie, P. F.-E., & Lips, R. A. (2010). Is there really a problem with hiring rural social service staff? An exploratory study among social service supervisors in rural Minnesota. *Families in Society, 91,* 433–439.

McBride, T., & Kemper, L. (2009, June). *Impact of the recession on rural America: Rising unemployment leading to more uninsured in 2009* (RUPRI Center for Rural Health Policy Analysis Brief No. 2009-6). Retrieved from http://www.

unmc.edu/ruprihealth/Pubs/b2009-6%20Rising%20Unemployment%20 Leading%20to%20More%20Uninsured.pdf

McNichol, E., Oliff, P., & Johnson, N. (2012). *States continue to feel recession's impact.* Retrieved from Center on Budget and Policy Priorities website: http://www. cbpp.org/cms/index.cfm?fa=view&id=711

Mossakowsky, K. N. (2008). Is the duration of poverty and unemployment a risk factor for heavy drinking? *Social Science and Medicine, 67,* 947–955.

National Association of Social Workers. (2009). *Social workers speak on the economy, April 2009.* Washington, DC: Author. Retrieved from http://www.naswdc.org/ pressroom/2009/sweconomiccrisis.pdf

National Association of Social Workers, Center for Workforce Studies. (2006). *Assuring the sufficiency of a frontline workforce: A national study of licensed social workers.* Retrieved from http://workforce.socialworkers.org/studies/ nasw_06_execsummary.pdf

Program Development and Evaluation. (2005). *Using the retrospective post then-pre design* (Quick Tips #27). Madison, WI: University of Wisconsin-Extension.

Reardon, C. (2009). Economic squeeze – The recession's impact on behavioral health. *Social Work Today, 9*(2), 12. Retrieved from http://www.socialworkto-day.com/archive/031109p12.shtml

Riebschleger, J. (2007). Social workers' suggestions for effective rural practice. *Families in Society: The Journal of Contemporary Social Services, 88,* 203–213.

Slovak, K., Sparks, A., & Hall, S. (2011). Attention to rural populations in social work scholarly journals. *Journal of Social Service Research, 37,* 428–438.

State of Hawai'i Department of Health. (2012). *State of Hawai'i Department Primary Care Needs Assessment Databook, 2012.* Retrieved from http://hawaii.gov/ health/doc/pcna2012databook.pdf

State of Hawai'i Department of Labor and Industrial Relations. (2009). *Occupational employment and wages in Hawai'i, 2008.* Honolulu, HI: Research and Statistics Office, State of Hawai'i Department of Labor and Industrial Relations.

Thomas, S. (2011, October 24). Hawai'i's jobless rate up 3.6 points since recession began. *Pacific Business News.* Retrieved from http://www.bizjournals.com/ pacific/news/2011/10/24/hawaiis-jobless-rate-up-36-points.html

U.S. Bureau of the Census. (2012, May). *2010 Census urban and rural classification and urban area criteria.* Retrieved from http://www.census.gov/geo/www/ ua/2010urbanruralclass.html

Vorsino, M. (2009, December 27). Hawai'i's welfare numbers rising for the first time in a decade. *Honolulu Advertiser.* Retrieved from www.staradvertiser.com.

Vorsino, M. (2010a, June 20). On O'ahu, crime up: Major offenses rise islandwide, prompting neighbors to unite in community watch and patrols. *Honolulu Advertiser.* Retrieved from www.staradvertiser.com.

Vorsino, M. (2010b, September 17). Poverty in Hawai'i highest since '97: Poor economic conditions have left more than 156,000 people in a struggle to make ends meet. *Honolulu Advertiser.* Retrieved from www.staradvdertiser.com.

Wu, C.-F. (2011, January). *Effects of the economic downturn on child support orders and payments.* Paper presented at the meeting of the Society for Social Work and Research Conference, Tampa, FL.

Better Together: Expanding Rural Partnerships to Support Families

HARRIET SHAKLEE

University of Idaho, Moscow, Idaho

JERI BIGBEE

University of California, Davis, California

MISTY WALL

Boise State University, Boise, Idaho

Chronic shortages of health, social service, and mental health professionals in rural areas necessitate creative partnerships in support of families. Cooperative extension professionals in Family and Consumer Sciences and community health nurses, who can bring critical skills to human services teams, are introduced as trusted professionals in rural communities. Multidisciplinary prevention programs offer particularly good contexts for county extension educators and community health nurses to work in collaboration with social workers. The case of grandparents raising grandchildren illustrates the critical roles that can be filled by professionals in these two fields to extend the reach of family support programs.

Rural and frontier areas experience chronic shortages of health, mental health, and social work clinicians. Sixty-six percent of areas federally designated as mental health profession shortage areas are rural. Particularly limited are those specializing in services to children and older adults (National Advisory Committee on Rural Health and Human Services [NACRHHS], 2008). A 2004 workforce survey found that 80% of social workers who work with children and adolescents serve in urban areas, whereas just 3% work in rural communities (Center for Health Workforce Studies, 2006). Given these limitations in access to mental health professionals in rural areas, it is not surprising that use of mental health services is lower in rural than urban areas (Gamm, Stone, & Pittman, 2003).

Research findings suggest that the social service needs of rural families are just as great, if not greater, than those of urban families. Studies consistently show poverty to be a strong risk factor for children, and poverty is particularly pronounced for rural children. The most negative child outcomes are found in areas of persistent poverty, where 20% or more of residents are in poverty for at least 30 years. Eighty-eight percent of areas of persistent poverty in the United States are in rural counties (NACRHHS, 2008).

Substance abuse is also more common in rural areas, starting in the teenage years and continuing through adulthood (NACRHHS, 2007). Abuse of alcohol, methamphetamine, narcotics, and prescription painkillers are of particular concern. Nearly twice as many young adults (age 18–25) in rural areas abuse Oxycontin and methamphetamine, compared to urban age mates, and 48% of young adults in larger rural areas (population 20,000 or more) reported engaging in binge drinking, i.e., five or more drinks on a single occasion (Maine Rural Health Research Center, 2007). Yet there are fewer detox and treatment facilities per capita in rural than in urban areas (NACRHHS, 2007).

The American Psychological Association (2012) highlighted several indicators that many rural families are overstressed. Rural communities include sizeable populations who are at elevated risk for mental health concerns, especially older residents and people who are chronically ill. The National Behavioral Health Survey shows a significantly higher rate of major depression among rural populations, and suicide is the second leading cause of death in rural areas (American Psychological Association, 2012).

The recent influx of immigrants and refugees to some rural communities can also test the limits of rural human services. First-generation immigrants are often challenged to learn the language and ways of their new country, while human services professionals must learn to adjust their programs to better accommodate the traditions of the new arrivals. Refugee groups come to U.S. communities after extended periods of trauma and often require culturally sensitive social services and counseling (Martinez-Brawley, 2009).

The recession of 2007 to 2011 has further burdened rural social service programs. Tax revenues diminished as the employment rolls shrank, family purchasing power contracted, and property values declined, all major sources of public funds. As a result, government-based social services were targets of budget cuts, reducing programs for family support. Nonprofits dedicated to family well-being were threatened as well, as grant opportunities were curtailed and foundation endowments lost value (Gais, 2009; McDaid & Knapp, 2010; Wise, 2009).

Financial stress for programs was mirrored in stress for families, who struggled with job loss, reduced incomes, home foreclosures, forced moves, homelessness, and an inability to meet nutritional, health, and educational needs of family members (Shaklee & Brown, 2009). Economic downturn can result in a perfect storm for health and social services, as program resources shrink just as family needs grow.

Limited resources must be used carefully when need exceeds capacity, including leveraging existing resources by collaborating with allied organizations and professions. Multidisciplinary teams of mental health professionals are often employed to help communities stretch program resources (NACRHHS, 2005). One successful collaborative approach is the wraparound model, in which professionals from complementary social service and mental health disciplines come together to meet the varied needs of individual families (Carney & Buttel, 2003).

When resources are taxed to the limit, rural social workers may find that other trusted professionals in the community can further extend the reach of human service programs. County cooperative extension educators and community nurses are introduced as natural partners in promoting family well-being in rural communities.

COOPERATIVE EXTENSION

Each state has one or more universities designated as a land-grant institution, endowed by the Smith-Lever Act of 1914 with a mission to provide research-based practical information to the public. Over the past 100 years, the resulting cooperative extension system has established a strong presence in communities throughout the United States. With its historical roots in agriculture and rural concerns, extension programming is a particularly trusted resource in small towns and rural areas (U.S. Department of Agriculture [USDA], 2011).

The cooperative extension system operates extensive programs throughout the nation, supported by funds from the USDA in conjunction with state and county monies. Local university extension programming emanates from county or regional offices in response to community needs. Strong links to university research facilities and faculty keep county educators updated in content (USDA, 2011).

Most relevant to human services are the many county extension educators representing Family and Consumer Sciences (FCS), with its interdisciplinary approach to families. FCS extension educators lead evidence-based programs in family relations, parenting, home safety, youth development, 4-H, fitness, nutrition, health, and caregiver support. Extension educators translate research findings into practices that families can use on an ongoing basis. Target audiences include marginalized groups and new arrivals, as well as mainstays of the community. Programs are developed to accommodate the needs of limited-education and low-income audiences (Hill & Parker, 2005; USDA, 2011).

COMMUNITY HEALTH NURSING

Community health nurses are also natural partners for family support programming. Community health nursing is a specialty area that provides care to individuals, families, and communities, based on a strong health promotion and advocacy approach. Since the early 20th century, this area of nursing practice has a tradition of creatively and collaboratively addressing the needs of rural populations through such innovative programs as the Frontier Nursing Service and the Red Cross Rural Nursing Service (Bigbee & Crowder, 1985).

Today, community health nurses practice in a variety of community-based settings, including public health departments, community clinics, schools, and home health/hospice agencies. An increasing percentage of nurses work in community health settings (as opposed to hospitals), particularly in rural and frontier areas. Like extension educators, nurses enjoy strong respect and trust among rural community residents (Bigbee, 1993).

Community health nurses and cooperative extension professionals share common perspectives and approaches, and collaboration between the groups can be particularly productive (Condo & Martin, 2002; Gray, 1990; Hall et al., 2005; Jenkins, 1991). One such nursing–extension collaboration in an isolated rural Idaho county integrated programs in health, safety, and family support (Bigbee, Hampton, Blanford, & Ketner, 2009). The authors concluded that "unlike some other practice settings, interdisciplinary cooperation is the norm in rural and frontier communities, based on the culture of strong community ties, the importance of social capital, and the need to maximize limited resources" (Bigbee et al., 2009, p. 196). From this perspective, a partnership between social workers, nurses, and cooperative extension professionals would be a logical extension of this "better together" rural ethic in addressing the human service needs of rural populations during challenging economic times.

PREVENTION MODELS AND MULTIDISCIPLINARY COALITIONS

Research has amply documented the effectiveness of prevention strategies in working with at-risk families, in areas as diverse as child abuse prevention, school engagement, and teen pregnancy prevention (see Bugenthal et al., 2002; Goldberg, Frank, Bekenstein, Garriety, & Ruiz, 2011; Prinz, Sanders, Shapiro, Whitaker, & Lutzker, 2009; Scribano, 2010, for example studies). Prevention programs work with families who evidence risk factors of concern, but have not yet shown the problematic behavior. Prevention programs are widely distributed among populations at risk (e.g., single parent, poverty-level income, high school dropout), rather than focusing on the smaller pool of families who actually develop the problem behaviors (e.g., family violence or substance abuse). Because consequences can be so severe and treatment so intensive for children and adults in families who exhibit dysfunctional behaviors, the more broadly based prevention strategies are often cost-effective, with more positive outcomes for families (DeBoard, 2005).

Current research also supports an integrated mental-plus-physical health approach, based on several studies showing that family life stressors compromise later physical as well as mental health outcomes. For example, the stresses of child abuse and neglect have been linked to indicators of poor physical health well into adulthood, in addition to the mental health concerns more traditionally linked to early abuse (Campbell, Greeson, Bybee, & Raja, 2008; Lanier, Jonson-Reid, Stahlschmidt, Drake, & Constantino, 2010; Maniglio, 2010). Such findings demonstrate the broad potential impact of effective family violence prevention programs and underscore the importance of collaboration between physical health and mental health programs under a shared human services umbrella.

Although prevention approaches to family support have a proven record of effectiveness in family support, resource limitations may undermine the capacity of rural social service agencies to extend their reach to prevention strategies. However, strategic collaborations with allied professionals in the community can allow human services programs to provide these critical support programs to stressed families.

MULTIDISCIPLINARY PREVENTION STRATEGIES

Prevention approaches to family well-being reach beyond traditional generalist and clinical social work strategies in engaging families. In particular, major components of prevention are educational and motivational. Families may need to reshape a problem pattern of behavior toward habits more likely to yield their desired outcomes. For example, positive discipline strategies may more effectively promote the achievement success a mother would like her child to experience, so that she will need to forego a family tradition of spanking in favor of alternative approaches. Program challenges include communicating information effectively so the mother understands it, working with her on a behavior change strategy, as well as motivating her to make the change.

These are challenges well explored by research in adult education, replete with evidence on learning styles and strategies that more readily translate into enduring behavior change. Adult education approaches are also careful to engage the learner as teacher, through a more egalitarian teaching relationship that shows respect for the life experience of adult learners. This style is naturally more culturally sensitive, as the teacher takes cues from the learner about family traditions and values (Merriam & Brockett, 1996).

County extension educators bring their content expertise to the educational setting, so that some may specialize in nutrition or fitness, whereas others teach about family relations and parenting. However, extension educators in general, regardless of content expertise, have learned effective strategies to engage adult learners in transformational learning (USDA, 2011). Adult learning is the specialty skill extension educators can bring to family support partnerships, complementing the talents and training of social workers and other human services professionals.

Strong extension ties to land-grant university campuses can bring other resources to a multidisciplinary human services team. Many social service programs have outstanding front line staff, but few resources for research and evaluation. However, continued access to tax dollars or grant funds depends on strong evidence of program effectiveness. FCS extension educators can link programs to evaluation and data analysis expertise on campus to provide affordable, high-quality program evaluation. Student engagement in such projects has added value, inspiring young adults' further interest in the human services and in small town and rural communities, and drawing future professionals to this area of critical need.

Like social workers and extension educators, community health nurses bring much-needed expertise to multidisciplinary family support teams. Many family support issues are evidenced in health outcomes, such as the compromised health of a malnourished child, or unexplained injuries from a violent home. Other family challenges stem from health issues, such as the difficulties of caring for a special needs child, or the resultant poverty when medical bills overtax family income.

Health services frequently serve as the front door to social services, as families reveal needs in the context of a health care visit. Health care settings can provide a neutral ground for families in need, particularly when working with known and trusted health professionals. Community-based nurses have the added advantage of their neighborhood-based family contacts, and the informal network of information they garner about family needs in the community.

Considering their extensive family needs, rural communities require strategic partnerships to provide the broadest possible network of support with limited resources. The potential power of a broad-based family support coalition is explored through the example of grandparents raising grandchildren, a family form in strong evidence in rural America (Bigbee, Musil, & Kenski, 2010).

COMMUNITY PARTNERS AND GRANDPARENTS RAISING GRANDCHILDREN

Family crisis can necessitate out-of-home placements to protect children. A parent's long-term physical or mental illness, substance abuse, incarceration, death, or military deployment may require that children be cared for by others. Most commonly, children are cared for by kin in informal arrangements made outside of the formal welfare system. For example, in Idaho in 2008 there were nine children in informal care with relatives for every one child in the foster care system (Shaklee, Bigbee, & Wall, 2008). Families are the first line of defense in times of family crisis.

Most frequently, grandparents are the ones who step into the parenting role, caring for 59% of children in the United States living with kin. In fact, one in 10 grandparents has been responsible for raising one or more grandchildren at some point in their lives, with rates even higher among African American and Hispanic populations (Fuller-Thomson & Minkler, 2005; Green, 2003; Hayslip & Kaminski, 2005). About one-third of U.S. grandparents raising grandchildren are older than age 60, 30% are not married, 30% have a disability, and nearly 20% live in poverty (Hayslip & Kaminski, 2005; Shaklee et al., 2008), all risk factors that point to a need for multifaceted support for these families in transition.

Most relatives raising their kin are thrust into the role with little warning, when a family crisis comes to a head. A return to childrearing may necessitate major life changes (Letiecq, Bailey, & Porterfield, 2009), including work roles (e.g., returning to work to earn more income, or quitting work to take care of the children), housing (e.g., moving to a larger space to accommodate the children, or looking for less expensive space to free up funds for children's expenses), and family finances (e.g., extending family income to provide children's food, clothing, and child care).

Major transitions in family structure come with emotional and social costs as well. Many grandparents lose their social networks when they take grandchildren into their homes and report frustration with the loss of freedom and adult friendship (Hayslip & Kaminski, 2005). Others are stressed as they navigate social service and legal systems in meeting family needs. Continued conflicts with the children's parents complicate the lives of grandparents raising grandchildren, along with frayed relationships with other family members. Family stress appears to be greatest in the first year of transition, with the quality of relationship with the grandchild mediating the course of the long-term adjustments for caregiving grandparents (Goodman, 2012; Letiecq et al., 2009).

The children in need of grandparent care often pose special challenges for their caregivers. Many of these children have lived in disorganized homes for years, with little parental guidance. Some have experienced prenatal exposure to drugs or alcohol as well. Family violence, neglect, poor nutrition, and irregular school attendance are common for children in need of out-of-home care. These life patterns may contribute to maladaptive behavior, attachment issues, poor school performance, mental illness, youth risk taking, substance abuse, and complex medical needs (Dubowitz et al., 1992; Dubowitz, Zurvin, & Star, 1993; Hayslip, Shore, Henderson, & Lambert, 1998; Musil, Warner, Zauszniewski, Wylke, & Standing, 2009).

All of these areas of challenge add up to a disruptive life for grandparenting families. A recent 6-month health intervention pilot study with seven rural families raising grandchildren found these significant stressors among the grandchildren, grandparents, and children's parents: diagnoses of childhood diabetes, elevated high school drop out rate, hospitalization, surgery, death, job loss, drug use, arrest, incarceration, and divorce (Bigbee, Vander Boegh, Prengaman, & Shaklee, 2011). A prevention-oriented family support strategy can help stressed families such as these avoid burn-out and maintain their effectiveness in meeting family needs.

Despite the challenges for children and grandparents, evidence suggests that kinship care may be the best resolution to a difficult situation for children. When parents are not able to fulfill their parental role, grandparents and other kin offer several advantages in child placement. Children living with relatives have more residential stability than those in foster placement with nonrelatives, a factor associated with more positive outcomes for children. The children report feeling less stigma in the homes of relatives than those with nonrelatives (Pabustan-Claar, 2007; Simms, Dubowitz, & Szilagyi, 2000). In addition, children in kinship placements are able to have more frequent and regular visits with biological parents, maintain ties with siblings, experience fewer placement changes, and preserve racial and cultural ties (Green, 2003; Metzger, 2008).

In sum, grandparents and other kin have become the dominant refuge for children in crisis. The transitional issues for grandparents and children point to a need for family support, but the nature of the family arrangements means that traditional social service providers may not have access to these families. Most caregiving grandparents are not formally designated foster parents, and the children's moves to their grandparents' homes take place outside of the social service system. In fact, caregiving grandparents commonly express fear of the social service system, concerned that they will lose the children to "the system," or become ensnarled in costly legal custody proceedings (Leticq et al., 2009). Under these circumstances, grandparenting families frequently pass under the radar of social service agencies.

Community nurses and extension educators may be able to serve as the gateway to family support for grandparents raising grandchildren. County extension educators are familiar with a broad sector of the community, particularly in small towns and rural areas. Health professionals are also tuned into family circumstances, particularly community health nurses with their extensive community ties. The health needs of aging community members also bring grandparents into frequent contact with health care providers. Working in established coalitions alongside social work and mental health professionals, FCS extension professionals and community nurses can connect stressed grandparenting families to available resources in the community. The success of multidisciplinary coalitions in supporting these families points to the viability of this approach (Ganthavorn & Hughes, 2007; Miller, Bruce, Bundy-Fazioli, & Fruhauf, 2010).

These coalitions are also in a position to develop programs specifically to meet the needs of caregiving grandparents. Those grandparents who feel isolated from their former network of friends may find support from the grandparent support groups available in many communities, often sponsored by cooperative extension programs. The children involved may find friendship in their new community through the 4-H programs offered through the extension office (Ganthavorn & Hughes, 2007; Miller et al., 2010).

Extension fitness and nutrition programs may also meet the needs of grandparents, who find they need more energy for their new responsibilities. Fitness activities can moderate stress experienced by grandparents as they work out the many adjustments to their new family form. The children in their care are relying on them for support for years to come, underscoring the importance of maximizing health outcomes when aging seniors return to the parenting role.

Health interventions have proven helpful to grandparents raising grandchildren. Home visitation programs targeting improved health have shown positive effects on physical, mental, and emotional health (Bigbee et al., 2011; Kelley, Whitley, & Campos, 2010). A program of health promotion, such as these for grandparents raising grandchildren, fits well with the mission and expertise of community health nursing and extension educator professionals and may be beyond the scope of work of most generalist social work practitioners.

This discussion demonstrates the power of an expanded human services partnership to support overstressed rural families, using the illustrative case of grandparents who take grandchildren into their homes. A multidisciplinary approach to family support including strategic cooperation among extension programs, community health nurses, and social workers can extend the reach of overburdened social service systems, maximize service delivery, and stimulate positive family outcomes. This strategy can be especially effective in rural and small town communities, where cooperative extension and community nursing have such long roots in the community, and can provide a natural complement to social work philosophy and practice.

REFERENCES

American Psychological Association. (2012). *The critical need for psychologists in rural America*. Retrieved from http://www.apa.org/about/gr/education/rural-need.aspx

Bigbee, H., Musil, C., & Kenski, D. (2010). The health of caregiving grandmothers: A rural–urban comparison. *Journal of Rural Health, 27,* 289–296.

Bigbee, J. (1993). The uniqueness of rural nursing. *Nursing Clinics of North America, 28*(1), 131–144.

Bigbee, J., & Crowder, E. (1985). The Red Cross rural nursing service: An innovative model of public health nursing delivery. *Public Health Nursing, 2*(2), 109–121.

Bigbee, J., Hampton, C., Blanford, D., & Ketner, P. (2009). Community health nursing and cooperative extension: A natural partnership. *Journal of Community Health Nursing, 26*(4), 192–197.

Bigbee, J., Vander Boegh, B., Prengaman, M., & Shaklee, H. (2011). Promoting the health of frontier caregiving grandparents: A demonstration project evaluation. *Journal for Specialists in Pediatric Nursing, 16,* 156–161.

Bugenthal, D., Ellerson, P., Lin, E., Rainey, B., Kokotovic, A., & O'Hara, N. (2002). A cognitive approach to child abuse prevention. *Journal of Family Psychology, 16*(3), 243–258.

Campbell, R., Greeson, M., Bybee, D., & Raja, S. (2008). The co-occurrence of childhood sexual abuse, adult sexual assault, intimate partner violence, and sexual harassment: A mediational model of posttraumatic stress disorder and physical health outcomes. *Journal of Consulting and Clinical Psychology, 76*(2), 194–207.

Carney, M., & Buttell, F. (2003). Reducing juvenile recidivism: Evaluating the wraparound services model. *Research on Social Work Practice, 13,* 551–568.

Center for Health Workforce Studies. (2006). *Licensed social workers in behavioral health, 2004.* Retrieved from http://workforce.socialworkers.org/studies/behavioral/behavioral_chap4.pdf

Condo, E., & Martin, K. (2002). Health professions and cooperative extension: An emerging partnership. *Journal of Extension, 40*(4), 4FEA2.

DeBoard, K. (2005). Communicating program value of family life and parenting education programs to decision makers. *Journal of Extension, 43*(2), 2IAW2.

Dubowitz, H., Feigelman, S., Zuravin, S., Tepper, S., Davidson, H., & Lichenstein, R. (1992). The physical health of children in kinship care. *American Journal of Diseases in Children, 146,* 603–610.

Dubowitz, H., Zurvin, S., & Star, R. (1993). Behavior problems of children in kinship care. *Journal of Developmental and Behavioral Pediatrics, 14,* 386–393.

Fuller-Thomson, E., & Minkler, M. (2005). American Indian/Alaskan Native grandparents raising grandchildren: Findings from the Census 2000 supplementary survey. *Social Work, 50*(2), 131–139.

Gais, T. (2009). Stretched net: The retrenchment of state and local social welfare spending before the recession. *Publius, 39*(3), 557–579.

Gamm, L., Stone, S., & Pittman, S. (2003). Mental health and mental disorders—A rural challenge: A literature review. In *Rural healthy people 2010* (pp. 97–114). College Station, TX: Southwest Rural Health Research Center.

Ganthavorn, C., & Hughes, J. (2007). Promoting healthy lifestyles among grandparents raising grandchildren in Riverside County. *Journal of Extension, 45*(1), 1FEA6.

Goldberg, B., Frank, V., Bekenstein, S., Garriety, P., & Ruiz, J. (2011). Successful community engagement: Laying the foundation for effective teen prevention. *Journal of Children and Poverty, 17*(1), 65–86.

Goodman, C. (2012). Caregiving grandmothers and their grandchildren: Well-being nine years later. *Children and Youth Services Review, 34,* 648–654.

Gray, M. E. (1990). Factors related to practice of breast self-examination in rural women. *Cancer Nursing, 13*(2), 100–107.

Green, R. (2003). *Kinship care, making the most of a valuable resource.* Washington, DC: Urban Institute Press.

Hall, C., Wimberly, P., Hall, J., Pfriemer, J., Hubbard, E., Stacy, A., & Gilbert, J. (2005). Teaching breast cancer screening to African American women in the Arkansas Mississippi River Delta. *Oncology Nursing Forum, 32*(4), 857–863.

Hayslip, B., Shore, J., Henderson, C., & Lambert, P. (1998). Custodial grandparenting and the impact of grandchildren with problems on role satisfaction and role meaning. *Journal of Gerontology: Social Science, 53B*(3), 164–173.

Hayslip, T., & Kaminski, P. (2005). Grandparents raising their grandchildren: A review of the literature and suggestions for practice. *The Gerontologist, 45,* 262–269.

Hill, L., & Parker, L. (2005). Extension as a delivery system for prevention programming: Capacity, barriers, and opportunities. *Journal of Extension, 43*(1), 1FEA1.

Jenkins, S. (1991). The future of rural communities: Mobilizing local resources. In A. Bushy (Ed.), *Rural nursing* (Vol. 2, pp. 16–28). Newbury Park, CA: Sage.

Kelley, S., Whitley, D., & Campos, P. (2010). Grandmothers raising grandchildren: Results of an intervention to improve health outcomes. *Journal of Nursing Scholarship, 42*(4), 379–386.

Lanier, P., Jonson-Reid, M., Stahlschmidt, M., Drake, B., & Constantino, J. (2010). Child maltreatment and pediatric health outcomes: A longitudinal study of low-income children. *Journal of Pediatric Psychology, 35*(5), 511–522.

Letiecq, T., Bailey, S., & Porterfield, F. (2009). "We have no rights, we get no help." The legal and policy dilemmas facing grandparent caregivers. *Journal of Family Issues, 29*(8), 995–1012.

Maine Rural Health Research Center. (2007). *Substance abuse among rural youth: A little meth and a lot of booze* (Research and Policy Brief). Retrieved from muskie.usm.maine.edu/Publications/rural/pb35a.pdf

Maniglio, R. (2010). The impact of child sexual abuse on health: A systematic review of reviews. *Clinical Psychology Review, 29*(7), 647–657.

Martinez-Brawley, E. (2009). "The world is flat": Is US rural social work flattening too? *Rural Society, 19,* 286–288.

McDaid, D., & Knapp, M. (2010). Black-skies planning? Prioritising mental health services in times of austerity. *British Journal of Psychiatry, 196,* 423–424.

Merriam, S., & Brockett, R. (1996). *The profession and practice of adult education: An introduction.* San Francisco, CA: Jossey-Bass.

Metzger, J. (2008). Resiliency in children and youth in kinship care and family foster care. *Child Welfare, 87*(6), 115–140.

Miller, J., Bruce, A., Bundy-Fazioli, K., & Fruhauf, C. (2010). Community mobilization model applied to support grandparents raising grandchildren. *Journal of Extension, 48*(2), 2IAW7.

Musil, C., Warner, C., Zauszniewski, M., Wylke, M., & Standing, T. (2009). Grandmother caregiving, family stress and strain, and depressive symptoms. *Western Journal of Nursing Research, 31*(3), 389–408.

National Advisory Committee on Rural Health, & Human Services. (2005). *The 2005 report to the secretary: Rural health and human service issues.* Retrieved from http://www.hrsa.gov/advisorycommittees/rural/2005secreport.pdf

National Advisory Committee on Rural Health, & Human Services. (2007). *The 2007 report to the secretary: Rural health and human service issues.* Retrieved from http://www.hrsa.gov/advisorycommittees/rural/2007secreport.pdf

National Advisory Committee on Rural Health, & Human Services. (2008). *The 2008 report to the secretary: Rural health and human service issues.* Retrieved from http://www.hrsa.gov/advisorycommittees/rural/2008secreport.pdf

Pabustan-Claar, J. (2007). Achieving permanence in foster care in young children: A comparison of kinship and non-kinship placements. *Journal of Ethnic and Cultural Diversity in Social Work, 16*(2), 61–94.

Prinz, R., Sanders, M., Shapiro, C., Whitaker, D., & Lutzker, J. (2009). Population-based prevention of child maltreatment: The U.S. Triple P system population trial. *Prevention Science, 10*(1), 1–12.

Scribano, P. (2010). Prevention strategies in child maltreatment. *Current Opinion in Pediatrics, 22*(5), 616–620.

Shaklee, H., Bigbee, J., & Wall, M. (2008). *Grand families count in Idaho, Idaho Kids Count.* Retrieved from www.idahokidscount.org/downloads/library/downloads/primary_research/Grand%20Families%20Count%20in%20Idaho.pdf

Shaklee, H., & Brown, J. (2009). *Small faces in a big recession, Idaho Kids Count: Quantitative report.* Retrieved from www.idahokidscount.org/downloads/library/downloads/primary_research/Small-Faces/SmallFacesPart1.pdf

Simms, M., Dubowitz, H., & Szilagyi, M. (2000). Health care needs of children in the foster care system. *Pediatrics, 106*, 909–918.

U.S. Department of Agriculture. (2011). *About us: Extension.* Retrieved from http://www.csrees.usda.gov/qlinks/extension.html

Wise, P. (2009). Children of the recession. *Archives of Pediatric Adolescent Medicine, 163*(11), 1063–1064.

Index

Note: Page numbers in **bold** type refer to figures
Page numbers in *italic* type refer to tables

INDEX